D0760827

Essential Dental Public Health

Blánaid Daly

Richard G. Watt

Paul Batchelor

Elizabeth T. Treasure

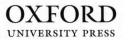

OXFORD

UNIVERSITY PRESS

OXFORD

UNIVERSITY PRESS

Great Clarendon Street, Oxford OX2 6DP

Oxford University Press is a department of the University of Oxford.
It furthers the University's objective of excellence in research, scholarship,
and education by publishing worldwide in

Oxford   New York
Auckland   Bangkok   Buenos Aires   Cape Town   Chennai
Dar es Salaam   Delhi   Hong Kong   Istanbul   Karachi   Kolkata
Kuala Lumpur   Madrid   Melbourne   Mexico City   Mumbai   Nairobi
São Paulo   Shanghai   Taipei   Tokyo   Toronto

Oxford is a registered trade mark of Oxford University Press
in the UK and in certain other countries

Published in the United States
by Oxford University Press Inc., New York

© Oxford University Press 2002

The moral rights of the author have been asserted

Database right Oxford University Press (maker)

First published 2002

A catalogue record for this book is available from the British Library

Library of Congress Cataloging in Publication Data
(Data available)

ISBN 0 19 262974 3

10 9 8 7 6 5 4 3 2 1

Typeset by Expo Holdings, Malaysia
Printed in Great Britain
on acid-free paper by T. J. International Ltd.

Foreword

Aubrey Sheiham, Professor of Dental Public Health, University College London.

Dentistry exists to help attain the highest level of oral health for all people at best, or the amelioration of dental pain and the improvement of oral functioning at least. It continues to deserve to exist only as long as it continues, or aspires, to meet such goals. Eighty years ago, Pickerill said this about dentistry: 'If during the past one hundred years, half as much time, money and brain power had been spent on the prevention of dental caries as had been spent on the perfecting of ways and means of replacing artificially tissue lost by disease there can be no doubt that the present condition of affairs would not have come about.' Unfortunately Pickerill's words are still relevant today. Relatively little emphasis is placed on effective dental public health and consequently high levels of dental disease and dental pain and functional disability are common. The main emphasis remains 'replacing artificially tissue lost by disease' despite the fact that no disease has ever been treated away and dental diseases are no exception. The limitations of conventional dentistry are serious. Therefore, on humanitarian grounds alone, a major shift to effective dental public health approaches are essential.

Dental diseases are the most common chronic diseases, and the mouth is the most expensive part of the body to treat in some countries. The persistence of high levels of dental diseases despite the availability of a scientific epidemiological basis for preventing them suggests that alternative approaches using public health principles, as outlined in this book, are needed. Dentistry is based on the implicit assumption that treatment and clinic-based prevention of disease by dentists would achieve better health and that resources would be available to fund their efforts. Sadly, even in Scandinavian countries with many dentists, dental diseases are still common and progressive. Dentistry has not been capable of controlling, nor effectively or efficiently preventing diseases. In an era of evidence-based public health medicine and dentistry, such approaches are no longer acceptable. Strategies should take into consideration that the major contribution to improving oral health falls outside conventional dental practice. Even if dentists were successful at treating disease in individual patients, for every patient treated successfully there will be many others developing disease because the determinants have not been addressed. The current approach is equivalent to dentists and their teams mopping the mess on the floor with better and more efficient mops, whilst leaving the tap full on. So the mess persists and may get worse and affect the underlying structures. Then more costly treatments are needed to remedy the accumulated destruction. A more rational solution is to try to turn the tap off and clean up the smaller mess that remains. That is, dealing with the determinants of the diseases and treating what remains effectively.

Health care systems embody our responses to perceptions of need. Dental thinking has been largely concerned with dentist-defined needs of individuals. This has shaped dental ethics (responsibility for the dentally diseased/sick), research questions ('Why do individuals develop caries?), and the planning of services. This thinking extends into risk identification and disease prevention: trying to identify individuals with high caries risk and concentrating efforts on them. The aim of that approach is to help the vulnerable minority and to reduce inequalities in health. Such a perspective may be commendable in humanistic terms, but it cannot solve the problem of a mass disease such as caries, which is progressive and occurs throughout the lifespan. The strategy is symptomatic, not radical. It does not attack the main determinants of caries. Those whom we particularly want to help represent the extreme of a continuous distribution of risks and behaviours. Therefore effective prevention requires changes that involve the population as a whole. The radical strategy for populations is to identify and if possible remedy the underlying causes of the causes of major dental health problems.

What alternative approaches are needed? A public health approach should include the following: a population, rather than a high-risk preventive strategy, a common risk-factor approach to prevention, and an intersectoral health promotion multi-level strategy. In addition, an evidence-based approach should be mandatory.

An organized, concerted population policy is needed to tackle the determinants based on contemporary concepts of health promotion. The high prevalence of dental caries is definitely related to sugars, therefore an important focus for prevention should relate to diet and to behaviour change. The environment determines behaviour. The most effective way to change behaviour is to change the environment within which people live, making healthy choices the easier choices and unhealthy choices more difficult. Such a policy is enabling and supportive.

Greater emphasis must be given to the development of upstream interventions because many of the risks for disease and poor health functioning are shared by large numbers of people. One-to-one interventions do little to alter the distribution of disease in the populations, because new people continue to be afflicted even as 'sick' people are treated or cured. It is therefore more cost-effective to prevent many chronic diseases using a common risk-factor approach at the community and environmental levels than to address them at the individual level.

The future of dental practitioners lies in advising patients about risks to dental health, investigating and controlling the risks, influencing the behaviour of patients, diagnosing oral and dental diseases and assessing patients' needs based on a combination of normative and perceived needs, providing high-quality evidence-based dental care – doing the right thing and doing it right, and lastly, administration of a dental team. Most dental practitioner involvement in dental public health policy development will be as health advocates. To increase effectiveness, advocates build partnerships with the community, other professional groups, and other sectors. They place their skills at the disposal of the community. Being on tap not on top.

Understanding and adopting the principles of dental public health described in this text should be considered as essential as knowing the principles of clinical procedures. I endorse what Roy Duckworth, the dean of a leading dental school, wrote in 1974 in the first British textbook of dental public health: 'Teaching community dentistry, ... should form the very hub of dental education around which its biological, clinical, and technological spokes should revolve.' Incorporating the principles outlined in this book will enable dentists to fulfill their professional and civic roles as altruistic health workers and encourage trust and personal satisfaction because they have done their best.

REFERENCES

Duckworth, R. (1974). Dental education. In *Dental public health* (ed. G. L. Slack and B. A. Burt), p. 293. Bristol, Wright.
Pickerill, H. P. (1923). *The prevention of dental caries and oral sepsis* (3rd edn). London, Baillière Tindall and Cox.

Preface

Dental public health is a recognized core subject in most undergraduate dental curricula. Dental students are required to cover a wide range of subjects in their undergraduate training. Dental public health is, however, quite different from many of the other basic dental sciences and clinical subjects within the crowded curriculum. Dental public health focuses upon the broader picture at a population level. It seeks to understand and explore the factors determining oral health and the most effective ways of preventing and treating oral diseases, and reducing inequalities. It encourages students to develop analytical skills and a questioning approach to the delivery of dental care. As health professionals, it is essential that dentists are equipped with the appropriate knowledge, skills, and values required to perform their role in society. Dental public health provides a key link between different subjects within the dental curriculum and developments in the health system more generally.

This book is designed for busy dental undergraduates. The text aims to provide an overview and introduction to the core elements of dental public health. Four sections cover the fundamental principles of public health, epidemiology, health promotion, and heath services. It is not possible to cover all of these subjects in great depth within one text; instead, this book presents an essential guide to each area. A range of tables, figures, and discussion points are presented to summarize and stimulate debate and discussion. Updates on dental service developments and other relevant information will be posted on the Oxford University Press website (http://www.oup.co.uk/isbn/0–19–262974–3). Key issues raised by the discussion points will also be posted on this website.

We hope you will find this an interesting and challenging read. In addition to the references listed, recommendations on further reading are also provided for those interested in further their understanding of this subject.

Blánaid Daly
Richard G. Watt
Paul Batchelor
Elizabeth T. Treasure

Permissions

Chapter 1

Fig. 1.2 Snow's map of cholera cases in Soho, 1854. Reproduced from Naidoo and Wills (2000) *Health Promotion: foundations for practice*, with permission from London, Balliere-Tindall).

Chapter 2

Fig. 2.1 The role of health care in reducing mortality. (a) Respiratory tuberculosis: death rates, England and Wales. (b) Whooping cough: death rates of children under 15, England and Wales. (c) Measles: death rates of children under 15, England and Wales.
Reproduced from McKeown and Lowe (1974), *An Introduction to Social Medicine*, with permission from Blackwell Science Ltd.

Fig. 2.2 Mortality trends, 1841–1985, England and Wales. The Standardized Mortality Ratio (SMR) is an index which allows for differences in age structure. Values above 100 indicate higher mortality than in 1950–52, and values below 100 indicate lower mortality.
Information borrowed from: Harrison D, Integrating health sector action on the social and economic determinants of health. Reviews of Health Promotion and Education Online: Verona Initiative, 1998. URL: http://www.rhpeo.org/iihp-articles/c-proceedings/verona/l/index.]itm with the authorization of the Editor in chief of RHPEO.

Fig. 2.3 Determinants of health. Dahlgren and Whitehead devised a diagram to show the general factors that affect health.
Source: based on Dahlgren, G. *European Health Policv Conference: opportunities,for the future. Volume II–Intersectoral action for health.* Copenhagen, WHO Regional Office for Europe, 1995.

Fig. 2.4 The widening mortality gap between social classes. Standardized Mortality ratios, indexed to 1930–32. Reproduced from Department of Health (1999) *Saving Lives: our healthier nation 1999*, Crown Copyright materials reproduced with permission of the controller of HMSO and Queen's Printer.

Fig. 2.5 The common risk-factor approach.
Reproduced with permission from Sheiham, A. and Watt, R. (2000). The common risk factor approach: a rational basis for promoting oral health. *Communitv Dentistry and Oral Epidemiologv*, 28, 399-406. O 2000 Munksgaard International Publishers Ltd. Copenhagen, Denmark.

Chapter 3

Fig. 3.1 Conceptual model of oral health.
Reproduced with permission from Locker, D. (1988). Measuring oral health: a conceptual framework. *Community Dental Health*, 5, 3–18 Copyright 2000 FDI World Dental Press Limited, London, UK

Chapter 4

Fig 4.2 Schematic models of four possible relationships between exposure to a cause and the associated risk of disease.
Reproduced from Rose (1992) *The strategy of preventive medicine* with permission from Open University Press.

Fig. 4.3 A hypothetical normal distribution of a disease within a population.
Reproduced from Ashton and Seymour (1988) *The new public health* with permission from Open University Press.

Chapter 5

Fig. 5.2 The conceptual model of health, adapted from WHO 1980. Reproduced with permission from Locker, D. (1988). Measuring oral health: a conceptual framework. *Community Dental Health*, 5, 3–18 Copyright 2000 FDI World Dental Press Limited, London, UK.

Chapter 6

Table 6.1 Proportions, past and projected, of adults with 21 or more standing teeth by age, rate of change with cohorts.
Reproduced with permission from Downer (1991). Improving dental health of United Kingdom adults and prospects for the future. *British Dental Journal*, **170**, 154–8. Copyright 1991 British Dental Journal, 64 Wimplole Street, London, WIM 8AL, UK

Table 6.2 Total decay experience of 5-year-old (dmft) and 8-, 12-, and 14-year-old children (DMFT) in England and Wales in 1973, 1983, and 1993 (weighted means), with proportions caries free.
Reproduced with permission from Downer (1994). The 1993 national survey of children's dental health: a commentary on the preliminary report. *British Dental Journal*, **176**, 209–14. Copyright 1994 British Dental Journal, 64 Wimplole Street, London, WIM 8AL, UK

Chapter 7

Box 7.1 Hierarchy of evidence.
Modified from Greenhalgh 1997. Reproduced with permission from Fig. 7.1 The process of using EBD to make clinical decisions.
Reproduced from Richards and Lawrence (1995). Evidence based dentistry. *British Dental Journal*, **179**, 270–273, with permission from the BMJ Publishing Group
Table 7.1 Framing a question.
Modified from Sackett (2002): UK Cochrane website. © Adapted from Sackett *et al.*, *Evidence Based Medicine*, 1996, by permission of the publisher Churchill Livingstone

Chapter 8

Box 8.4 Broad fields of research.
Modified from Greenhalgh (1997). How to read a paper: getting your bearings. *BMJ*, **315**, 243–246. Reproduced with permission from the BMJ Publishing Group

Chapter 9

Fig. 9.1 Ottawa Charter for health promotion.
Reproduced with permission from WHO 1986. *The Ottawa Charter for Health Promotion*. Health Promotion 1. iii–v. Geneva. WHO.
Fig. 9.2 The common risk-factor approach.
Reproduced with permission from Sheiham, A. and Watt, R. (2000). The common risk factor approach: a rational basis for promoting oral health. *Community Dentistry and Oral*

Epidemiology, 28, 399-406. © 2000 Munksgaard International Publishers Ltd. Copenhagen, Denmark.

Chapter 10

Fig. 10.1 The health belief model.
Reproduced from Becker and Maiman (1975). *Medical care* with permission from Lippincott Williams and Wilkins.

Fig. 10.2 Diffusion of innovation.
Reproduced from Becker and Maiman (1975). *Medical care* with permission from Lippincott Williams and Wilkins.

Chapter 11

Fig. 11.1 A flowchart for Planning and evaluating health education. Reproduced from Ewles and Simnett 1999 with permission from Harcourt Publishers Ltd.

Chapter 12

Fig. 12.1 Classification of Sugar (Reproduced from Watt 1999 with permission copyright HMSO).

Fig. 12.2 Changing patterns of sugar consumption in the UK, 1942–96.
Reproduced with permission from Sustain: The alliance for better food and farming, (2000), *Sweet and sour–The impact of sugar production and consumption on people and the environment*, Sustain, London (www.sustainweb.org).

Fig. 12.3 Advertising budgets on sugars.
Reproduced with permission from Sustain: The alliance for better food and farming, (2000), *Sweet and sour–The impact of sugar production and consumption on people and the environment*, Sustain, London (www.sustainweb.org).

Chapter 15

Fig 15.1 Incidence rates of oral cancer by deprivation, 1986–95. (Reproduced from CRC Cancerstart report, with permission from the Cancer Research Campaign)

Fig. 15.2 Age standardised mortality rates for male cancer of the lip, tongue, mouth and pharynx, England and Wales, 1911–98. (Reproduced from CRC Cancerstart report, with permission from the Cancer Research Campaign)

Fig. 15.3 Relative risk of oral/pharyngeal cancer in males by alcohol/tobacco using US measures. (Reproduced from CRC Cancerstart report, with permission from the Cancer Research Campaign)

Fig 15.4 Smoking cessation protocol. (Reproduced with permission from Watt and Robinson 1999 with permission copyright HMSO)

Chapter 21

Fig. 21.1 Rational Planning model (Reproduced from McCarthy 1982 with permission from King's Fund)

Fig. 21.3 Quality assurance cycle.
© Reprinted from *Promoting Health* (Ewles and Simnett), 1992, by permission of the publisher Bailliere Tindall.

Chapter 22

Fig. 22.1 Age- and sex-adjusted mortality rates for the United States (1900-73) (including and excluding eleven major infectious diseases) contrasted with the proportion of Gross National Product expended on medical care.

Reproduced with permission from McKinlay and McKinlay (1977). The questionable contribution of medical measures to the decline in mortality in the United States in the twentieth century. *MMFQ*, **55**, 406–28.

Fig. 22.2 Comparative analysis of alternative courses of action in economic evaluation. © Michael F. Drummond, Bernie J. O'Brien, Greg L. Stoddart and George W. Torrance, Second Edition, 1997. Reprinted from *Methods for the Economic Evaluation of Health Care Programmes* by Michael F. Drummond, Bernie J. O'Brien, Greg L. Stoddart and George W. Torrance (Second Edition, 1997) by permission of Oxford University Press.

Fig. 22.3 Measurement of costs and consequences in economic evaluation. © Michael F. Drummond, Bernie J. O'Brien, Greg L. Stoddart and George W. Torrance, Second Edition, 1997. Reprinted from *Methods for the Economic Evaluation of Health Care Programmes* by Michael F. Drummond, Bernie J. O'Brien, Greg L. Stoddart and George W. Torrance (Second Edition, 1997) by permission of Oxford University Press.

Chapter 23

Box 23.4 The determinants of health inequality.
Whithead, 'The concepts and principles of equity and health'. The determinants of heath inequality. *Health Promotion International*, **Vol. 6**, 1991, pp. 217–226, by permission of Oxford University Press.

Fig. 23.1 Model of access.
Reproduced from Department of Dental Public Health 2001 Kings College London with permission.

Contents

Contents

Authors

Dr Paul Batchelor Senior Lecturer and Honorary Consultant in Dental Public Health, Eastman Dental Hospital, University College London, Bloomsbury Campus, 1–19 Torrington Place, London WC1E 6BT and Research Director, Centre for Dental Services Studies, Department of Health Sciences, Alcuin Teaching Building, University of York, Heslington, YO10 5DD. paulb@public-health.ucl.ac.uk

Ms Blanaid Daly Lecturer, Dept of Dental Public Health and Oral Health Services Research, GKT Dental Institute, Denmark Hill Campus, Caldecot Road, SE5 9RW. blanaid.daly@kcl.ac.uk

Professor Elizabeth T. Treasure, Professor and Honorary Consultant, Dental Public Health Unit, The Dental School, Heath Park, Cardiff CF14 4XY, Wales. TreasureET@cardiff.ac.uk

Dr Richard G. Watt, Reader, Royal Free & University College Medical School, University College London, Bloomsbury Campus, 1–19 Torrington Place, London WC1E 6BT. r.watt@ucl.ac.uk

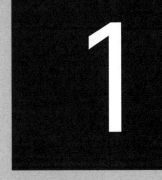

Principles of
dental public health

1 Introduction to the principles of public health

CONTENTS

By the end of this chapter you should be able to:

- Define dental public health.
- Identify the links between clinical practice and dental public health.
- Outline the criteria used to determine if a condition is a public health problem.
- Describe the central arguments presented by the critiques of the biomedical approach to health care delivery.

This chapter links with:
- All the other sections in this text by providing the background to dental public health.

INTRODUCTION

Public health is now recognized as being a core component of the undergraduate medical and dental curricula (General Dental Council 1997; General Medical Council 1993). This recognition acknowledges that public health is an important subject relevant to the practice of medicine and dentistry. This chapter will outline what is meant by public health and, in particular, its relevance to clinical dental practice. The philosophical and historical background of public health will be reviewed and the limitations of the traditional system of health care highlighted. Finally, a dental public health framework will be outlined to highlight the central importance of public health to the future development of dentistry.

DEFINITION OF DENTAL PUBLIC HEALTH

Dental public health can be defined as the science and practice of preventing oral diseases, promoting oral health, and improving quality of life through the organized efforts of society.

The science of dental public health is concerned with making a diagnosis of a population's oral health problems, establishing the causes and effects of those problems, and planning effective interventions. The practice of dental public health is to create and use opportunities to implement effective solutions to population oral health and health care problems (Chappel *et al.* 1996).

Dental public health is concerned with promoting the health of the population and therefore focuses action at a community level. This is in contrast

Table 1.1 Stages of clinical and public health practice

Individual clinical practice	Public health practice
Examination	Assessment of need
Diagnosis	Analysis of data
Treatment planning	Programme planning
Informed consent for treatment	Ethics and planning approval
An appropriate mix of care, cure, and prevention	Programme implementation
Payment for services	Types of finance
Evaluation	Appraisal and review

Modified from Young and Striffler 1969.

to clinical practice which operates at an individual level. However, the different stages of clinical and public health practice are broadly similar (Table 1.1).

Dental public health is a broad subject which seeks to expand the focus and understanding of the dental profession on the range of factors that influence oral health and the most effective means of preventing and treating oral health problems. Dental public health is underpinned by a range of related disciplines and sciences which collectively enrich the value and relevance of the subject (Box 1.1)

RELEVANCE OF PUBLIC HEALTH TO CLINICAL PRACTICE

The practice of dentistry is undergoing a period of rapid change due to a wide range of factors in society (Box 1.2). The knowledge and skills required for the next generation of dental professionals will therefore be very different than was previously the case.

Box 1.1 Sciences and disciplines underpinning dental public health

- Epidemiology
- Health promotion
- Medical statistics
- Sociology and psychology
- Health economics
- Health services management and planning
- Evidence-based practice
- Demography

Box 1.2 Changes affecting the practice of dentistry

Epidemiological changes Changing pattern of disease; for example, dramatic improvements in caries, persistence of oral health inequalities.

Demographic shifts Ageing population, changes in family structures, greater population mobility, increasing cultural diversity.

Organizational changes NHS reforms, greater emphasis on primary care services and prevention, evidence-based medicine/dentistry, corporate bodies, clinical governance.

Professional development Importance of life-long learning, team work, interpersonal skills.

Social change Consumerism, increasing public expectations and demands on health services, widening social and economic inequalities.

Political pressures Changes to the welfare state, pressures for cost containment on public spending, rationing care, increasing professional accountability.

Technological change Health informatics, pharmaceutical developments, 'new genetics', new dental materials.

Studying dental public health provides an ideal opportunity to gain an improved understanding of many of the factors outlined above. Three key areas are most relevant to the practice of clinical dentistry, as detailed below.

Epidemiology of oral diseases

It is essential that dental services are developed to address and effectively meet the oral health needs of individuals and the wider community. Knowledge of the epidemiology of oral disease will facilitate an understanding of the extent, aetiology, natural history, and impacts of oral conditions. By applying critical appraisal skills in their clinical decision-making, dental professionals can practice dentistry more effectively through an evidence-based approach to care. Clinical epidemiology provides the skills required to undertake this task by teaching the principles of study design and evaluation.

Prevention and oral health promotion

Prevention is as pivotal to the dentist's role as treatment of disease. A core aspect of dental public health is exploring the principles of prevention and oral health promotion and identifying opportunities for effective preventive interventions. This requires an understanding of the social, political, economic, and environmental factors that influence oral health and the capacity of dentistry to influence them. Of particular importance to oral health is a broad understanding of diet and nutrition, body hygiene, tobacco use, and the use of fluorides in the prevention of dental caries, periodontal disease, and oral cancers.

Planning and management of health services

Dental services are a part of the health care system and are affected by many of the complex organizational and policy developments of the wider health, social, and welfare systems. It is essential that dental professionals have a broad understanding of the changing structure, organization, and finance of their health care system. This knowledge will enable dentists to plan and develop their dental practices more effectively.

WHAT IS A PUBLIC HEALTH PROBLEM?

It is now widely recognized that demands on health care systems will always be greater than the resources available to meet these needs. This dilemma is not confined to the developing world where resources are acutely limited. The richest countries in the world, such as the USA, Germany, and the UK are faced with similar problems of increasing demands and escalating health care expenditure. For example, expenditure on health care in the USA rose from 3.6% of gross domestic product in 1929 to 13.6% in 1995, and there is a prediction that it may reach 20% in the next few decades (Burt and Eklund 1999). In the UK spending on the General Dental Services has risen steadily over recent years. In 1977/78 the figure was £270 million and by 1997/98 the figure was £1528 million, a six-fold increase over a 10-year period (Dental Practice Board 1998).

DISCUSSION POINTS

What factors contribute to the increasing demands on health care systems? Are there any ways in which this demand can be controlled?

One response to increasing demands and limited resources is to direct resources to particular problem areas. However, what would be considered an important problem? This is where core public health principles have a major contribution to make. Box 1.3 lists certain public health criteria that can be used to determine the significance of a health problem (Sheiham 1996).

Box 1.3 Criteria for a public health problem

• Prevalence of the condition.
• Impact of the condition on an individual level.
• Impact on wider society.
• Condition is preventable and effective treatments are available.

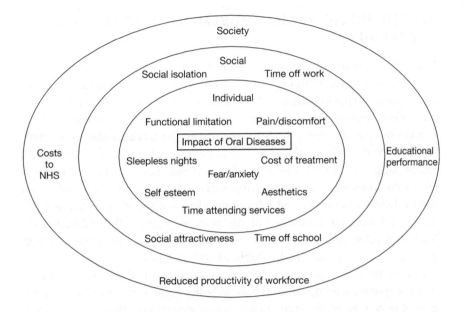

Fig. 1.1 The impact of oral disease.

The first criterion relates to the prevalence of the health problem, in essence is the disease widespread? Who has the disease? What percentage of the total population is affected? What is the distribution of the disease within the community? Is the prevalence of the condition increasing or decreasing? The second aspect relates to the impact of the condition at the individual level. How severe are the effects of the disease to the patient? For example, do people die as a result of it? Do they suffer pain, discomfort, or loss of function? Can they perform their normal social roles? Are they prevented from going to school or becoming employed because of the problem? The third aspect relates to the effects of the disease across society. What are the costs to the health service of treating the condition? How much time do people take off work to get treatment and care? What effect does the condition have on economic performance and productivity of the country? Figure 1.1 presents a summary of the impact of oral conditions on the individual and society. Finally, it is important to consider the potential for prevention and treatment of the disease. Is the natural history of the disease fully understood? Can the early stages of the condition be recognized? If so, are there interventions that can implemented to stop the disease progressing? If it does progress, are there effective treatments available?

DISCUSSION POINTS

Apply the above criteria to dental caries, periodontal disease, and malocclusion. Do you consider these oral health conditions are dental public health problems? Explain the basis for your answer.

BRITISH PUBLIC HEALTH MOVEMENT: HISTORY AND BACKGROUND

Public health is not a new subject. Indeed, it has a long and interesting history, which is linked to many of the social, economic, and political changes that have occurred in British history in the last 150 years. The public health movement originally arose in response to the appalling living and working conditions that affected a high proportion of the working classes in nineteenth century Britain. Rapid industrialization and urban growth created industrial towns in which overcrowding, extreme poverty, squalor, and disease were commonplace. Pioneering social reformers such as Southwood Smith, Edwin Chadwick, and John Snow identified the need to improve the living and working conditions of the poor to promote the public health. Municipal reforms and improvements in the environment then resulted from passing legislation such as the Public Health Act 1875.

One example of this early public health approach to dealing with disease is the response to a cholera outbreak in Soho, London in 1875. John Snow, a local doctor, identified that cholera was a waterborne disease by mapping the outbreak to a single water source, a water pump in Broad Street. By removing the pump handle, the epidemic was controlled as no one could then access the infected water source (Fig. 1.2). An example of public health practice in action: an epidemiological assessment of the problem, identification of the environmental cause of the infection, and implementation of effective action, cheaply and quickly.

DISCUSSION POINTS

- If John Snow had not been in Soho, how would this cholera outbreak have been dealt with by his less enlightened colleagues?
- What would have been the obvious limitations of this approach?

Public health reforms that focused upon improving environmental conditions which significantly boosted the health of the poor in Victorian and Edwardian Britain were not simply driven by altruistic motives. The need for a fit and healthy workforce and armed services were the main pressures for reform. A significant proportion of army recruits for the Boer War were rejected on health grounds, many of them because of dental problems. It was reported that 6% of potential recruits were rejected because of missing or decayed teeth and within 3 months of enlisting, 3 in every 1000 soldiers were declared unfit because of dental problems (Gelbier 1994).

The industrial revolution and the development of mechanization influenced emerging ideas about health and disease. The lessons of the public health movement were overtaken by the growth of knowledge about the

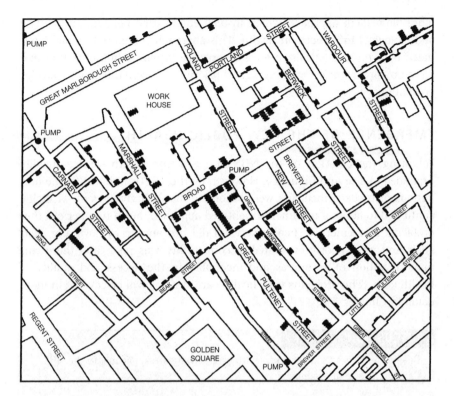

Fig. 1.2 Snow's map of cholera cases in Soho, 1854. (Reproduced from Naidoo and Wills 2000, with permission from Balliere-Tindall. See Permissions.)

functioning of the body and the analogy of the body with machines. The engineering concept was easy to explain to lay people, but it focused health interventions on the individual rather than the population level. This approach became known as the biomedical model of health. Features of the biomedical model are presented in Box 1.4.

By the turn of the twentieth century the focus of public health had shifted away from social and environmental causes of disease to a

---

Box 1.4 Features of the biomedical model

- Disease orientated, with a focus on pathological change.
- Explanations for ill health concentrate on biological factors, operating at an individual level.
- Knowledge and expertise controlled by the medical profession.
- Compartmentalized and mechanistic approach to diagnosis and treatment.
- Interventionist and high-technology approach to treatment – belief in 'magic bullets'.
- Top-down approach – hierarchical structure.
- Centralized institutional centres of excellence – teaching hospitals.

more biomedical approach which instead emphasized behavioural lifestyle and biological influences on health. This approach therefore became dominated by a more medicalized form of practice in which immunization and screening programmes had the highest priority and were the major focus for prevention.

EMERGENCE OF THE NEW PUBLIC HEALTH

Following the creation of the NHS in 1948, the health service steadily expanded in size and influence. However, by the 1970s and 1980s the limitations of modern medicine were becoming increasingly evident. Medicine continued to adopt a treatment-orientated approach, but a number of other problems also emerged: health services did not appear to have any clear goals and were poorly evaluated, accountability was poor, and there was maldistribution of resources and inequality in the access and quality of health care. (The problems with health care systems will be covered in more detail in Chapter 23.)

DISCUSSION POINTS

Do you think these problems of health care delivery are applicable to the NHS? Can you give some examples?

The limitations of modern medicine were highlighted by a selection of influential philosophers and academics whose criticisms of the current system of health care were very important in establishing the new public health movement. A synthesis of their main arguments are presented in Box 1.5.

The new public health movement has refocused attention on to the political, economic, and environmental influences on health within contemporary society. More emphasis is therefore placed upon developing a range of policy options to create a more health-promoting environment. This development requires health professionals to work collaboratively with a wide range of sectors and agencies. The improvement in health is largely dependent upon activities outside of the health services. This presents a major challenge to traditional beliefs of the role of medicine in society. A number of international reports and declarations embodied the new public health approach and the refocusing on primary health care. The most significant of these declarations was the Alma Ata Declaration.

ALMA ATA DECLARATION

In 1978 World Health Organization organized an international conference in Alma Ata in the then Soviet Republic of Kazakhstan to review the future

---

Box 1.5 Influential figures in the new public health movement

Archie Cochrane (1972)
Founder of the Evidence-Based Medicine movement. Identified lack of scientific evidence for large amount of clinical practice. Stressed need to evaluate all forms of medical care with randomized controlled trial. Also stressed the importance of the caring role in medicine.

Rene Dubos (1960)
Argued that modern society's obsession with the attainment of 'perfect health' was a 'mirage', an impossible dream. Instead proposed concept of holistic health as being a state of balance, equilibrium, and harmony with nature. Stressed the limitations of the doctrine of specific aetiology which dominates biomedical practice.

Ivan Illich (1976)
Major critique of modern medicine and medicalization of life. Stressed iatrogenic 'threat to health' of medical care. Concerned by power and control of medical profession in modern society and peoples' lack of autonomy in coping with life, illness, and death.

Thomas McKeown (1979)
Demonstrated that the major reductions in mortality in the nineteenth century were due to decline of infectious diseases. Main reasons for decline were improvements in nutrition, sanitation, water supply, and reduction in family size. Medical services and discoveries had relatively small effect. Stressed that if medicine is to be effective it should be concerned with prevention as well as treatment, with care as well as cure, and with the context of sickness as well as intervention.

Nancy Milio (1986)
A key figure in the field of health promotion. Coined the expression 'making the healthier choices the easier choices'. Reviewed the importance of healthy public policy and the importance of developing health alliances to promote health.

Geoffery Rose (1985)
A leading figure influencing the development of modern public health and preventive medicine. Outlined the limitations of the traditional high-risk strategy in preventive medicine and the potential advantages of the whole-population approach in disease prevention.

Vincente Navarro (1976)
Critical of the commercialization of health and the emphasis placed upon profit and financial gain. Stressed how the capitalist system has taken over health care as a commodity to be bought and sold. Also identified how the system defines diseases and formulates politically driven solutions that fail to challenge the underlying factors that create disease.

---

development of health care internationally (WHO 1978). The conference agreed an important declaration which has since set an agenda for the new public health:

Focus on prevention A shift in focus and resources is required, away from the dominant concentration on treatment towards prevention and what we now term as health promotion.

Multi-sectoral approach The promotion of health requires action in a wide range of sectors beyond the health sector. Education, agriculture, transport, economic, housing and welfare policies all affect health.

Appropriate technology Emphasis should be placed upon the most appropriate technology and personnel to deal with health problems.

Equitable distribution Governments and health planners must endeavour to fairly distribute those factors which influence health.

Community participation Individuals and communities should participate in all decisions which affect their health.

These concepts are fundamental to the core themes in dental public health practice.

CORE THEMES OF DENTAL PUBLIC HEALTH PRACTICE

Dental public health is a fundamental subject for dental students to study, but unlike the majority of subjects in the dental curriculum dental public health aims to broaden students' focus and encourage a critical and questioning approach to the delivery of dental care. This approach is based upon understanding and applying core public health themes to the delivery of dental care. These themes include:

Concepts of health

As health professionals, it is important that dentists have a clear understanding of what is meant by oral health. What dimensions would be included within a definition of oral health? Professional and public concepts may differ over the meaning and selected priorities. This may have important implications for the focus of dental services, goals, and priorities set, and the best process of evaluating interventions.

Determinants of health

To promote and maintain oral health, it is essential that the factors which determine the health status of individuals and populations are clearly identified and the appropriate action implemented. Public health research and policy analysis has highlighted the significance of social, economic, and environmental factors in determining health status, and the need to work collaboratively with the range of sectors which influence these factors. At the root of understanding the socio-environmental determinants is the practical concept that, in order to change people's behaviour, one has to change the environment.

Concepts of need

One of the greatest challenges facing health care systems internationally is meeting the health needs of their populations with the available resources. This complex political and clinical problem has firstly to consider how to define need. Bradshaw (1972) has developed a taxonomy that distinguishes four types of need.

Normative needs These are defined by professionals, based upon an assessment against an agreed set of criteria.

Felt needs These are the needs which people perceive as being important. They are subjective feelings of what people really want.

Expressed needs These arise from felt needs but are expressed in words or action and therefore become demands. People express a need when they ask for information or when they use services.

Comparative needs This is when an individual or group is compared with a similar individual or group and is considered lacking with regards to services or resources.

Inequalities in oral health

Within any given population, health will vary for a variety of reasons. Some health disparities may be considered acceptable when they are seen as being inevitable consequences of age or sex differences. Other health differences are caused by social, economic, and political factors which may affect certain members of society more than others purely based upon opportunity and access to appropriate resources within society. These health inequalities are now considered as unjust and unacceptable. The epidemiology of dental diseases reveals that disease levels vary greatly across socio-economic groups. What can dentists do to reduce oral health inequalities? One of the key challenges to dental public health is implementing effective strategies to do just this.

Preventive approach

Although 'prevention is better than cure', in reality prevention is given far less priority than the treatment of existing disease. Public health, however, seeks to develop effective preventive measures at both individual and population levels. Effective prevention requires an understanding of the key influences on health and identifying opportunities for appropriate intervention.

Quality of dental care

Although oral health is determined by a wide range of factors beyond purely contact with dental services, it is still important that high-quality dental services are developed to best meet the needs of their local populations. From a dental public health perspective quality of dental care encompasses a range of issues beyond solely clinical concerns. Issues such as access to care, responsiveness to individuals' concerns, and cost effectiveness all need to be addressed. Dental public health principles are relevant to clinical governance activities which encompass evidence-based dentistry.

Evidence-based practice

A core component of quality is the effectiveness of care. Evidence-based practice is central to clinical practice, and all clinical decisions should be based upon a critical appraisal of the available scientific evidence. Studying clinical epidemiology provides the understanding and skills to develop evidence-based practice.

IMPLICATIONS OF DENTAL PUBLIC HEALTH FOR PRACTICE, RESEARCH, AND TEACHING

The present UK government has placed public health at the centre of its health strategy (Department of Health 1999). Policies aimed at reducing health inequalities and addressing the social, economic, and environmental determinants of health are being developed and implemented. This public health agenda will directly impact upon the future development of dental services.

Dental public health is relevant to all aspects of clinical dental care, from the assessment of need, through the development of care, to the evaluation of treatment. The following chapters will introduce and explore the range of topics that are key elements of this subject.

REFERENCES

Bradshaw, J. S. (1972). A taxonomy of social need. In *Problems and progress in medical care*, Seventh series (ed. G. McLachlan), pp. 69–82. Oxford University Press.

Burt, B. and Eklund, S. (1999). Financing dental care. In *Dentistry, dental practice and the community*, 5th edn (ed.), pp. 89–114. Philadelphia, Saunders.

Chappel, D., Maudsley, G., Bhopal, R., and Ebrahim, S. (1996). *Public health education for medical students: a guide for medical schools*. Newcastle upon Tyne, University of Newcastle upon Tyne.

Cochrane, A. (1972). *Effectiveness and efficiency*. London, Nuffield Provincial Hospital Trust.

Dental Practice Board (1998). *Adult and child treatment GDS annual statistics 1977/78–1997/98*. Eastbourne, Dental Data Services.

Department of Health (1999). *Saving lives: our healthier nation*. London, The Stationery Office.

Dubos, R. (1979). *Mirage of health*. New York, Harper Colophan.

Gelbier, S. (1994). Where have we come from? In *Introduction to dental public health* (ed. M. C. Downer, S. Gelbier, and D. E. Gibbons), pp. 11–39. London, FDI World Press.

General Dental Council (1997). *The first five years: the undergraduate dental curriculum.* London, General Dental Council.

General Medical Council (1993). *Tomorrow's doctors: recommendations on undergraduate medical education.* London, General Medical Council.

Health Development Section (1999). *Promoting oral health 2000–2004: strategic directions and framework for action.* Melbourne, Public Health Division, Department of Human Services.

Illich, I. (1976). *Medical nemesis: the expropriation of health.* New York, Bantam Books.

McKeown, T. (1979). *The role of medicine.* Oxford, Basil Blackwell.

Milio, N. (1986). *Promoting health through public policy.* Ottawa, Canadian Public Health Association.

Naidoo, J. and Wills, J. (2000). *Health promotion: foundations for practice.* London, Baillière Tindall.

Navarro, V. (1976). *Medicine under capitalism.* London, Croom Helm.

Rose, G. (1985). *The strategy of preventive medicine.* Oxford, Oxford University Press.

Sheiham, A. (1996). Oral health policy and prevention. In *Prevention of oral diseases* (ed. J. Murray), pp. 234–49. Oxford, Oxford University Press.

WHO (World Health Organization) (1978). *Primary health care, Alma Ata 1978.* 'Health for All' Series no. 1. Geneva, WHO.

Young, W. and Striffler, D. (1969). *The dentist, his practice, and his community.* Philadelphia, Saunders.

FURTHER READING

Burt, B. A. and Eklund, S. (1999). *Dentistry, dental practice and the community.* Philadelphia, Saunders.

Downer, M. C., Gelbier, S., and Gibbons, D. E. (ed.) (1994). *Introduction to dental public health.* London, FDI World Press.

Murray, J. (ed.) (1996). *The prevention of dental disease* (3rd edn). Oxford, Oxford University Press.

Pine, C. (ed.) (1997). *Community oral health.* Oxford, Wright.

2 Determinants of health

CONTENTS

By the end of this chapter you should be able to:

- Describe the underlying range of factors that determine people's health.
- Outline the nature of, and explanations for, inequalities in health.
- Describe the basis for the common risk/health factor approach.
- Stress the importance of working in partnership with other agencies and organizations to promote health.

This chapter links with:

- Introduction to the principles of public health (Chapter 1).
- Definitions of health (Chapter 3).
- Public health approaches to prevention (Chapter 4)
- All chapters in the prevention and oral health promotion section (Chapters 9–16).

INTRODUCTION

For health services to deliver effective treatment and prevention a detailed understanding of the factors influencing health is critical. These factors are known as the determinants of health. Failure to address the underlying causes of disease in society will mean that sustainable improvements in the health of the population and a reduction in health inequalities will never be achieved. Tackling the contemporary determinants of health across society is a core function of public health and has now become the focus of government health policy (Department of Health 1999).

THE BROADER PICTURE

Many clinicians often feel frustrated when their advice to patients on ways of staying healthy is apparently ignored. Why don't people stop smoking when they know the serious health risks of the habit? Why do some parents continue to give their children sweets when they have been given clear advice on the harmful effects on the child's oral health? It is important for all health professionals to understand the factors influencing their patients' choices and actions. Clinicians equipped with this knowledge are more likely to be effective at supporting their patients and enjoying their professional work.

DISCUSSION POINTS

Peter is 18 years old and will soon be leaving school to study law at Oxford. He lives with his parents who are both accountants working in the City of London. They have a very comfortable standard of living. Peter is a confident, bright, and popular individual. His oral health is very good. He has only one filling and his oral hygiene is sound. He successfully completed a 3-year course of orthodontic treatment last year. He attends the family dentist on a regular basis.

Jane and Steve are both in their mid-twenties and have two children aged under 5 years. Steve left school with no qualifications and has never been able to find any permanent work. Jane has a part-time job in the local supermarket. Their oldest child, Britney, has had toothache for several weeks, and recently attended the local hospital where she had six teeth removed under a general anaesthetic. Both Jane and Steve are frightened of going to the dentist but are very anxious that their children should have good teeth.

Tom, a retired joiner, is 70, and lives in a council flat with his wife Mary. He has smoked for the last 55 years and enjoys the odd whisky with his mates. He is edentulous and has worn his present set of dentures for 6 years. For the last 9 months he has noticed a white mark on the side of his tongue but as this has not caused him any real pain or discomfort he hasn't bothered going to the doctor. He last saw a dentist when he had his dentures fitted.

List all the factors influencing these individuals' general and oral health?

Group these different factors under suitable subheadings.

How do these different factors relate to each other?

When asked what factors determine health, many people would probably highlight the importance of modern medicine. The use of antibiotics, high tech equipment, and surgical advances might all be given as the most important reasons for improvements in health that have been achieved in the last hundred years. Why is modern medicine credited with such achievements and is this a true reflection of reality?

Professor Thomas McKeown, a pioneer in public health research, conducted a detailed historical analysis of the reasons for the steady reduction in mortality rates that occurred in Westernized countries during the last century (McKeown 1979). In his classic analysis he investigated changes in mortality rates for different conditions. As can be seen in Fig. 2.1, with infectious diseases such as tuberculosis, whooping cough, and measles, significant reductions in mortality rates occurred long before treatments and vaccination programmes were introduced.

McKeown concluded that the most important reasons for the decline in mortality rates were social changes in society such as improvements in living conditions and sanitation, access to clean water, better nutrition, and reduced family size (McKeown 1979). Indeed, it has been claimed that medical treatments contributed only 17% to the gain in life expectancy that occurred in the twentieth century (Tarlov 1996). Figure 2.2 highlights that, by 1948 when the NHS was established, mortality rates had already declined greatly.

Modern medicine and dentistry have an important role to play in caring for people and improving their quality of life (McKeown 1979). However, the underlying importance of the social, economic, and environmental factors that determine the health of the population need to be recognized.

SOCIAL DETERMINANTS OF HEALTH

In many countries around the world, governments and the health professions are now increasingly acknowledging the importance of addressing the social determinants of health (WHO 2000). Public health research over the last 20 years has highlighted the impact on health of such factors as poverty, poor housing, unemployment, and social isolation (Marmot and Wilkinson 1999). Adverse conditions and influences can have a particularly significant effect at critical points in the life course (Bartley *et al.* 1997). Figure 2.3 presents an overview of the complex range of factors that determine the health status of individuals and populations.

DISCUSSION POINTS

Consider housing, one of the factors listed in Fig. 2.3. Describe the range of health problems that may be caused by poor housing.

LIMITATIONS OF THE LIFESTYLE APPROACH

Health professionals have traditionally focused upon changing the behaviours of their patients as the main means of promoting health and preventing disease, the so-called lifestyle approach. Smoking, alcohol and drug misuse, unsafe sex, poor eating, and a lack of exercise are all behaviours that are part of an individual's lifestyle. In the first list below, a series of recommendations for good health are presented by Professor Liam Donaldson, chief medical officer in England (Department of Health 1999). In contrast, the second list presents the recommendations for ways of staying healthy from an independent research unit (Townsend Centre for International Poverty Research 2000).

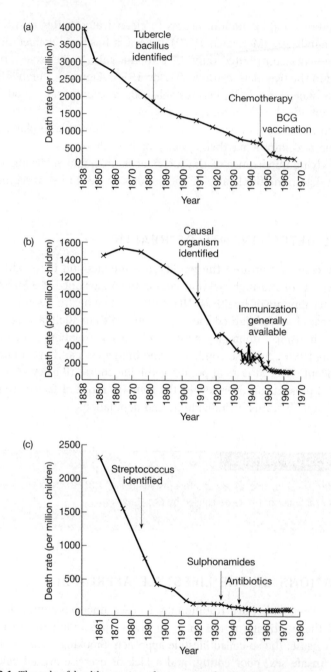

Fig. 2.1 The role of health care in reducing mortality. (a) Respiratory tuberculosis: death rates, England and Wales. (b) Whooping cough: death rates of children under 15, England and Wales. (c) Measles: death rates of children under 15, England and Wales. (Reproduced from McKeown and Lowe 1974, with permission from Blackwell Science Ltd. See Permissions.)

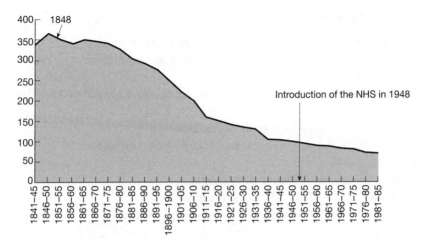

Fig. 2.2 Mortality trends, 1841–1985, England and Wales. The Standardized Mortality Ratio (SMR) is an index which allows for differences in age structure. Values above 100 indicate higher mortality than in 1950–52, and values below 100 indicate lower mortality. (Reproduced from Harrison 1998 with permission. See Permissions.)

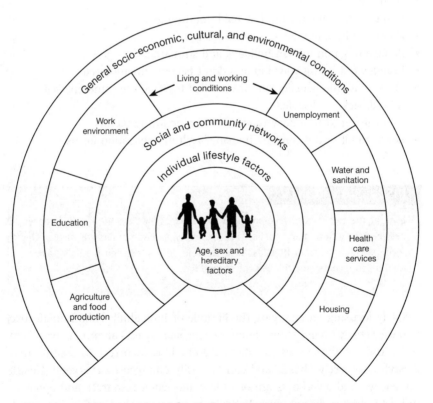

Fig. 2.3 Determinants of health. Dahlgren and Whitehead devised a diagram to show the general factors that affect health. (Based on Dahlgren, G., 1995. Reproduced with permission. See Permissions.)

Ten tips for better health

- Don't smoke. If you can, stop. If you can't, cut down.
- Follow a balanced diet with plenty of fruit and vegetables.
- Keep physically active.
- Manage stress by, for example, talking things through and making time to relax.
- If you drink alcohol, do so in moderation.
- Cover up in the sun, and protect children from sunburn.
- Practice safer sex.
- Take up cancer screening opportunities.
- Be safe on the roads: follow the Highway Code.
- Learn the first aid ABC: airways, breathing, circulation.

Ten tips for healthy living

- Don't be poor. If you can, stop. If you can't, try not to be poor for long.
- Don't have poor parents.
- Own a car.
- Don't work in a stressful, low paid, manual job.
- Don't live in damp, low-quality housing.
- Be able to go on foreign holidays and sunbathe.
- Practice not losing your job and don't become unemployed.
- Take up all the benefits you are entitled to, if you are unemployed, retired, sick, or disabled.
- Don't live next to a busy road or near a polluting factory.
- Learn to fill in the complex housing/asylum application forms.

DISCUSSION POINTS

Look at the two lists of recommendations above. What are the key differences between the different approaches? What underlying assumptions are made in the recommendations from Donaldson? What role do doctors and dentists have in relation to recommendations in the second list?

Solely focusing on changing the lifestyle of individuals is both ineffective and very costly (Syme 1996). Such an approach diverts attention away from the causes of the causes (Sheiham 2000). It is incorrect to assume that lifestyles are freely chosen and can be easily changed by everyone. Health knowledge and awareness are of little value when resources and opportunities to change do not exist. Behaviours are enmeshed within the social, economic, and environmental conditions of living (Graham 1999). Individuals' behaviours are therefore largely determined by the conditions in which they live (Sheiham 2000). Focusing solely on changing lifestyle can be considered a 'victim blaming' approach which is not only ineffective but may also widen health inequalities (Schou and Wight 1994).

HEALTH INEQUALITIES

What do we mean by inequalities in health? It would be unrealistic to expect everyone in society to have the same level of health. For example a teenager is far more likely to be physically fit than a man aged 75. Women may suffer from cervical cancer whereas this is obviously not a health problem for men. These differences are due to the effects of ageing or biology and are therefore unavoidable. Health inequalities refers to differences that are both avoidable and considered unacceptable in modern society.

In the UK research into health inequalities has largely focused upon the links between health and social class. The Black Report (Townsend and Davidson 1982) demonstrated that for almost all reported conditions the mortality and morbidity rates were higher in people from lower socio-economic groups. A follow up report, *The health divide* (Whitehead 1988), confirmed this finding and demonstrated that the gaps had actually increased. The most recent report has undertaken a comprehensive review of health inequalities (Acheson 1998). It found that although mortality has fallen over the last 50 years there are still substantial inequalities in health and that in some cases the differences have actually increased. The review considered that the evidence supported a socio-economic explanation of health inequalities. As a result it felt that underlying causes (the determinants) must be addressed. They pointed out that factors such as income, employment, and education, could not be affected by the Department of Health alone and stated that there was a need for a whole-government approach to dealing with the problems.

Health inequality is widespread: the most disadvantaged have suffered most from poor health. Box 2.1 lists the extent of health inequalities in modern Britain.

Box 2.1 The extent of inequalities in health

- Of the 66 major causes of death in men, 62 were more common among the lower social classes.
- Of the 70 major causes of death in women, 64 were more common in women from the lower social classes.
- A child born into a lower social class is twice as likely to die before the age of 15 as a child born into a higher social class.
- A man in a higher social class is likely to live around 7 years longer than a man in a lower social class.

(Department of Health 1996)

During the 1980s and 1990s the gap between the rich and the poor widened. Indeed the health gap now is considerably greater than in the 1930s (Department of Health 1999; Fig. 2.4).

Why do these inequalities exist? The Black Report outlined four possible explanations for health inequalities (Townsend and Davidson 1982).

Artefact That inequalities are not real, but rather a function of how social class and health are measured.

Selection process This explanation proposes that people in poor health drift down the social scale. Based upon this analysis, health therefore determines social class position.

Lifestyle effects The social distribution of risk behaviours such as smoking and drug misuse is higher amongst the lower social classes.

Materialistic and structuralistic factors This argument places emphasis upon the effects of poverty and disadvantage on health.

DETERMINANTS OF ORAL HEALTH

One of the problems with modern dentistry is the fact that it has become very isolated from other elements of the health service. However, when one

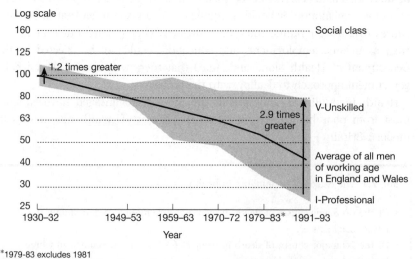

*1979-83 excludes 1981
England and Wales. Men of working age (varies according to year, either aged 15 or 20 to age 64 or 65)
Note: These comparisons are based on social classes I and V only.

Fig. 2.4 The widening mortality gap between social classes. Standardized Mortality Ratios, indexed to 1930–32. (From Department of Health 1999. Crown Copyright material reproduced with the permission of the Controller of HMSO and Queen's Printer. See Permissions.)

considers the issues raised in this chapter it should be very apparent that many of the points apply equally to both general and oral health. Indeed, from a public health perspective the importance of integrating oral health into the broader picture is critically important. For example, based upon McKeown's work, an analysis of the factors responsible for the improvements that have taken place in dental caries levels in many Westernized countries has revealed the relatively minor role played by dental services (Nadanovsky and Sheiham 1995).

DISCUSSION POINTS

Let's consider an oral health problem such as oral cancer. Based upon the issues raised in this chapter so far, describe the determinants of this condition. Attempt to draw a pictorial image of the various factors and how they relate to each other.

A contemporary understanding of the social determinants of health provides a basis for an integrated approach to preventing a range of conditions, the common risk-factor approach (WHO 2000). The fundamental basis of this approach is the importance of focusing attention on changing a small number of factors that determine a large number of diseases. Diet, smoking, alcohol, injury, hygiene, stress, and exercise are linked with a wide range of important diseases such as cancers, heart disease, and diabetes (Fig. 2.5). Altering these factors will reduce the risks of these systemic conditions as well as oral diseases such as caries, periodontal disease, and oral cancer (Sheiham and Watt 2000). Such an approach is likely to be more effective and efficient than traditional isolated disease-specific actions.

In addition to focusing action on the risk factors, this perspective also gives scope for promoting health factors that provide a supportive environment for good health and well-being. As a whole-population approach (see Chapter 4 for further details) inequalities in oral health can be reduced.

PARTNERSHIP WORKING

What role do health professionals have within this broader framework? Most do not have any direct influence over factors such as housing quality, government policy, or local planning decisions, but these factors clearly do have an effect on health. Therefore it is very obvious that health professionals need to work in partnership with a range of different organizations and agencies to effectively promote health. Working across professional boundaries is a challenging task which requires appropriate skills in communication and team working.

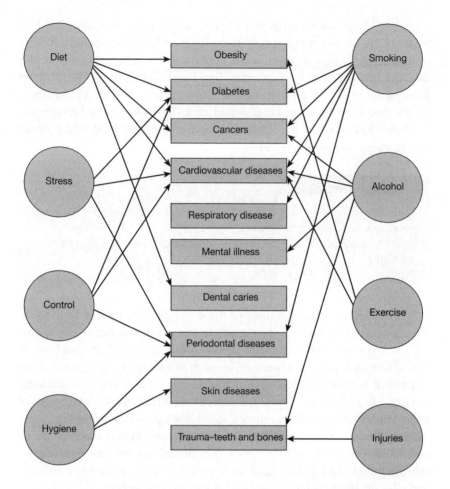

Fig. 2.5 The common risk-factor approach. (Reproduced from Sheiham and Watt 2000 with permission. See Permissions.)

DISCUSSION POINTS

To reduce smoking rates amongst young people, what agencies and organizations would have an important role to play?

A key task for public health professionals is to act as advocates for change to promote health and reduce inequalities. Advocacy involves influencing decision- and policy-makers to ensure that health is placed upon their agendas. A range of government initiatives have been launched in recent years to reduce health and social inequalities. A key to the success of these developments will be how effective the partnerships are in working together for sustainable change.

CONCLUSION

A fundamental issue of great importance to all health professionals is the need to identify and tackle the causes of disease in society. The promotion of health and a reduction in health inequalities requires effective action on the determinants of health. This chapter has given an overview of the social determinants of health and stressed the limitations of a lifestyle approach. The nature of, and explanations for, health inequalities have been presented. The importance of adopting an integrated approach to the promotion of oral health has been highlighted.

REFERENCES

Acheson, D. (1998). *Independent inquiry into inequalities in health: a report.* London, The Stationery Office.

Bartley, M., Blane, D., and Montgomery, S. (1997). Health and the life course: why safety nets matter. *British Medical Journal,* **314**, 1194–6.

Dahlgren, G. (1995). *European Health Policy Conference: opportunities for the future.* Copenhagen, WHO Regional Office for Europe.

Department of Health (1996). *Variations in health. What can the Department of Health and the NHS do?* London, HMSO.

Department of Health (1999). *Saving lives: our healthier nation.* London, The Stationery Office.

Graham, H. (1999). Promoting health against inequality – using research to identify targets for intervention: a case study of women and smoking. *Health Education Journal,* **57**, 292–302.

Harrison, D. (1998). Verona initiative: integrating health sector action on the social and economic determinants of health. *Internet Journal of Health Promotion:* http://www.monash.edu.au/health/IJHP/Verona

McKeown and Lowe (1974). *An Introduction to Social Medicine.* Oxford, Blackwell Science Ltd.

McKeown, T. (1979). *The role of medicine.* Oxford, Basil Blackwell.

Marmot, M. and Wilkinson, R. (ed.) (1999). *Social determinants of health.* Oxford, Oxford University Press.

Nadanovsky, P. and Sheiham, A. (1995). The relative contribution of dental services to the changes in caries levels of 12-year-old children in 18 industrialized counties in the 1970s and early 1980s. *Community Dentistry and Oral Epidemiology,* **23**, 231–9.

Schou, L. and Wight, C. (1994). Does health education affect inequalities in dental health? *Community Dental Health,* **11**, 97–100.

Sheiham, A. (2000). Improving oral health for all: focusing on determinants and conditions. *Health Education Journal,* **59**, 64–76.

Sheiham, A. and Watt, R. (2000). The common risk factor approach: a rational basis for promoting oral health. *Community Dentistry and Oral Epidemiology,* **28**, 399–406.

Syme, L. (1996). To prevent disease: the need for a new approach. In *Health and social organisation: towards a health policy for the 21st century* (ed. D. Blane, E. Brunner, and R. Wilkinson), pp. 21–31. London, Routledge.

Tarlov, A. (1996). Social determinants of health: the sociobiological translation. In *Health and social organisation: towards a health policy for the 21st century* (ed. D. Blane, E. Brunner, and R. Wilkinson), pp. 103–117. London, Routledge.

Townsend Centre for International Poverty Research (2000). *Ten tips for staying healthy.* London, UK Public Health Association.

Townsend, P. and Davidson, N. (1982). *Inequalities in health: the Black Report.* Harmondsworth, Penguin.

Whitehead, M. (1988). *The health divide.* London, Health Education Council.

WHO (World Health Organization) (2000). *Global strategy for the prevention and control of non communicable diseases.* Geneva, WHO.

FURTHER READING

Acheson, D. (1998). *Independent inquiry into inequalities in health: a report.* London, The Stationery Office.

Marmot, M. and Wilkinson, R. (ed.) (1999). *Social determinants of health.* Oxford, Oxford University Press.

3 Definitions of health

CONTENTS

By the end of this chapter you should be able to:

- Describe the concepts of health, disease, illness, and ill health from the perspective of a professional and a lay person.
- Outline the influence the concept of health may have on need and service use.
- Discuss how the gap between professional and lay concepts of health may have an impact on how health care is delivered, used, and evaluated.

The chapter links with:
- Determinants of health (Chapter 2).
- Overview of epidemiology (Chapter 5).
- Planning dental services (Chapter 21).
- Problems with health services (Chapter 23).

INTRODUCTION

In any discussion of public health it is necessary to be able to define what is meant by the term 'health'. The promotion and maintenance of health should be a goal of health services and thus a clear definition is essential. At a personal level we can distinguish the difference between feeling well and feeling ill, but converting this to an index that measures health and illness in a population is far more complex (Hart 1985). Health, disease, illness, and ill health mean different things to different people at different times, and providers of health care may hold very different views of health and illness to the users of health care, who have a lay perspective. This chapter will briefly review the commonly used definitions of health, disease, illness, and ill health, and will consider some of the implications these differences have for the measurement of health, the assessment of need, and how health care is delivered, used, and evaluated.

DEFINITIONS OF HEALTH, DISEASE, ILLNESS, AND ILL HEALTH

Health

Many attempts have been made to define health and to explore individuals' perceptions of the concept. After the Second World War, the WHO (1946) proposed a positive and holistic view of health:

> Health is a complete state of physical, mental and social well-being and not merely the absence of disease or infirmity.

DISCUSSION POINTS

Think back over the last year. Estimate how much of the time this description might have been applied to you. What were the factors that stopped you enjoying full health as outlined in this definition? Again thinking back over the last year, how would you rate your health compared with the rest of society? Is this a realistic definition of health? If not, why not?

The original WHO definition was criticized as being unrealistic, unworkable, and unachievable. Based upon this definition almost any defect or problem meant that a person would be considered 'not healthy'. The definition does, however, move beyond the concept that no disease is equivalent to health and that health has other dimensions beside the physical.

A pioneering French study (Herzlich 1973) identified that health was described in a variety of ways by lay people:
- As a state of being, and the absence of illness.
- As something to have, an inner strength or resistance to ill health.
- As a state of doing and being able to fulfil the maximum potential for life.

Blaxter (1990), based upon a review of the concept, had another description:

> Health can be defined negatively, as the absence of illness, functionally as the ability to cope with everyday activities, or positively, as fitness and well-being.

Ewles and Simnett (1999) have outlined the dimensions that they consider to be part of a complete view of health, termed 'a holistic concept of health', described in six separate areas (see Box 3.1).

It is very important to note that these areas are not separate but are in fact part of a whole. As you read this you may feel that not all of them apply to you as an individual. The importance of each is likely to vary at different times in your life. For example, the need to form social relationships is of

---

Box 3.1 The dimensions of health

1. Physical health: concerned with the functioning of the body.
2. Mental health: the ability to think clearly and coherently.
3. Emotional health: to recognize and express emotions such as fear, joy, grief.
4. Social health: to form and maintain relationships.
5. Spiritual health: concerned with either religious beliefs and practices or personal creeds and principles of behaviour.
6. Societal health: a person's health is closely linked to the environment he or she lives in.

(Modified from Ewles and Simnett 1999.)

---

particular importance when leaving home for the first time, while for the majority of people their physical health is of little concern at this time but becomes more so later in life.

So, modern concepts of health have moved from an 'absence of disease focus' to a concept that has a number of dimensions, and health has become defined in terms of social, psychological, and physical functioning (Reisine 1985). Health is a dynamic subjective concept which is influenced by an array of factors.

DISCUSSION POINTS

Outline the range of factors that determine how an individual would define their health.

A more recent WHO (1984) definition of health summarizes well the nature of contemporary understanding of the concept:

Health is the extent to which an individual or group is able, on the one hand to realize aspirations and satisfy needs; and on the other hand, to change or cope with the environment. Health is, therefore, seen as a resource for everyday life, not an object of living; it is a positive concept emphasizing social and personal resources, as well as physical capacities.

Disease

Disease can be described as named pathological entities diagnosed by means of clinical signs and symptoms, for example cancer or caries. Diseases are determined by professionals based upon information collected in history-taking and through clinical investigations and tests. The concept of disease has often been considered objective in nature; however, definitions of disease are not static and are also influenced by societal and cultural factors.

DISCUSSION POINTS

On a scale of 1 to 10, with 1 indicating most definitely a disease and 10 indicating the condition is most certainly not a disease, score the following conditions:

- Alcoholism
- Acne
- Gingivitis
- Gulf War Syndrome
- Hairy tongue
- Trans-sexuality
- Depression

Compare your scores with other members of your class.
What factors influenced your decisions?
What are some implications of the results of this exercise?

Illness

Illness refers to the subjective response of the lay individual to being unwell. It refers to how the person feels and what effect this has on their normal everyday life (Naidoo and Wills 1996).

Ill health

Illness and disease are clearly not the same. A person can have a disease and have no symptoms, for example, periodontal disease. However, if that person reports bleeding gums and loose teeth then they have symptoms and periodontal disease may be confirmed by evidence of attachment loss clinically and bone loss on radiographs. The disease and the illness coincide. Ill health is an 'umbrella term used to refer to the experience of disease plus illness' (Naidoo and Wills 1996).

DEFINITIONS OF NEED

The definition and concept of need is essential for planning and evaluation of oral health care (Sheiham and Spencer 1997). In relation to health, the concept of need may be divided into two aspects: the need for health care (the ability to benefit from health care) and the need for health (as described in the WHO definition of health) (Bowling 1997; Culyer 1976; WHO 1946).

Most discussions on the concept of health concentrate on the need for health care.

Different definitions of need have been proposed. In Chapter 1 Bradshaw's (1972) taxonomy of need was described. This definition is based on who defines the need. Carr and Wolfe (1979) describe another aspect of need which they term unmet need. This is the difference between the health judged to be needed and the health care actually provided. Cooper (1979) has suggested a taxonomy of need which is broadly similar to Bradshaw. See Box 3.2.

Box 3.2 Cooper's taxonomy of need

Wants   A person's own estimation of want for health.
Demand The wants an individual demands a professional to meet.
Need   A state judged as in need by a health professional.

(Modified from Cooper 1975)

Health care cannot meet all needs. This necessitates choices about what needs to meet and difficult decisions about whose needs will remain unmet.

PROFESSIONAL AND LAY PERSPECTIVES OF NEED

Most needs assessments are based on normative, or professionally defined need. The clinical indicators in current use do not take account of the individual's perception of need. So normative needs that are not of concern to the patient may be met. See the example in the following discussion point.

DISCUSSION POINTS

A complaint has been received about you by your local Health Authority as follows:

I went to the dentist because my teeth were crooked and I wanted them straightened, but what happened was the dentist filled a back tooth which had a hole that I didn't know about (which never troubled me) and then she told me I was too old for orthodontics.

(AW, aged 24)

Can you give an explanation for what has gone wrong between you and your patient?
How might it have been avoided?

Current clinical indicators only assess the physical signs of health and disease, yet this is only one aspect of a person's health state. Indicators in the future must therefore also include functional and psychological measurements (James 1999).

The gap between a lay person's (the patient's) perception of need and a professional's (the dentist's) perspective has been described as the 'clinical iceberg'. This is another important concept in relation to need. Many people may have undiagnosed serious disease or undiagnosed early disease which could be easily treated.

It could be supposed that symptoms that people experience which have not resulted in a visit to a health professional are mild, but this is not the case. Doctors are often not consulted for problems that have a successful treatment regimen. How and why people use services is related not only to the illness but also its symptoms and how the sufferer and others (e.g. friends and immediate family) respond to the symptoms. It is not possible to discuss all aspects in relation to perception of illness and service use here, however Scrambler's (1997) useful summary has been modified and is presented in Box 3.3.

DEFINITIONS OF ORAL HEALTH

Having considered the definition of general health, and the difficulties involved in so doing, how might we define oral health? Based on the WHO (1946) definition outlined above, we could define it as a completely healthy dentition (with 32 sound straight teeth and no periodontal or other soft tissue lesions) which results in 'a state of physical, mental and social well being'. But this is obviously impractical, unrealistic, and unachievable. A more appropriate definition might be 'a comfortable and functional dentition that allows individuals to continue their social role (Dolan 1993).

Locker (1988) has developed a conceptual model of oral health which defines health not only as an absence of disease but also includes functional aspects and social and psychological well-being. It provides a context in which to consider health, disease, impairment, disability, and handicap. By focusing on optimal functioning and social role, Locker's model addresses many of the limitations of normative clinical need assessment. It has provided the context for the development of oral health related quality of life measures (OHQoL) which are described in Chapter 21. The model and a brief explanation is reproduced in Box 3.4.

The definition of oral health may seem to be an irrelevant matter to the individual practitioner but it is worth considering what the effect might be if the definition of health were wrong. A definition sets the goal to which demands and treatments are aimed. If the definition is wrong then strategies to improve health or to provide health care will not achieve the most appropriate aims. The direction is likely to be inappropriate. This may lead

Box 3.3 Perception of illness and service use

Cultural variation
There is a marked cultural variation in how symptoms are interpreted. Some cultures will want to withdraw when in pain, other cultures will want to make a load noise and involve everyone.

Presentation of disease and knowledge of disease
Diseases which present dramatically often prompt service, for example toothache. However, the severity of the symptom does not imply serious disease. Many cancers have a slow insidious onset. People's decision to access care is related to their understanding of disease and their ability to distinguish between serious and not serious disease.

Triggers
People may have symptoms for a while before they choose to obtain care. Zola (1972) has described five key triggers: interpersonal crisis; interference with social or personal relationships; sanctioning (pressure from others to consult); interference with physical or vocational functioning, and temporalizing. This latter terms means setting a time related deadline: if the pain is not gone by the end of the weekend I shall go to the doctor.

Perceptions of costs and benefits
Are the benefits worth the cost of seeking care? Costs could relate to explicit costs such as patient charges for dental treatment and hidden costs such as transport, time off work, and child-care charges.

Lay referrals and intervention
Potential patients have a lay referral system. Symptoms are discussed with family, friends, and colleagues before a professional is accessed. Certain cultures who use an extended lay referral system may have low consultation rates. In other cases lay people may take it upon themselves to initiate an intervention if the symptoms are perceived to be serious (e.g. someone fitting in the street) or if the person is judged temporarily incapable (e.g. a parent for a child).

Geography and availability of services
It is acknowledged that health care is distributed in inverse proportion to need, termed the 'inverse care law' (Tudor Hart 1971). There are more doctors in middle-class areas than in socially deprived areas where the burden of illness is greater. If people perceive that services are not available, they do not demand care. Thus services continue to be poorly available (O'Mullane 1977). People who are homeless and people with learning difficulties often lack the resources, support, and skills to demand health care.

Self-care, self-help, and alternative therapies
Adults tend to use self medication as an alternative to going to the doctor.

(Modified from Scrambler 1997.)

Fig. 3.1 Conceptual model of oral health

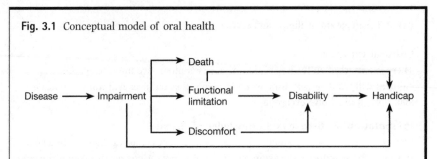

Fig. 3.1 Conceptual model of oral health. (Reproduced from Locker 1988 with permission. See Permissions.).

Impairment Anatomical loss, structural abnormality, or disturbance in chemical processes.
Functional limitation Restriction in the functions customarily expected of the body.
Pain and discomfort Self-reported pain and discomfort, physical and psychological symptoms, and other not-directly-observable feeling states.
Disability Limitations in, or lack of ability to perform, the activities of daily living.
Handicap The disadvantage and deprivation experienced by people with impairments. Functional limitations, pain, and discomfort or disabilities because they cannot or do not conform to the expectations of the group to which they belong.

(Reproduced with permission from Locker 1988. See Permissions)

to an over-ambitious service. If a strategy defines, for example, minor gingivitis as a condition that needs treatment, then the service will be directed towards this aim. The responsibility for this condition will be moved from the individual to the clinician. The service costs will increase and direction will be altered towards care for a very common disease with minimal long-term consequences.

However, adopting Dolan's definition may lead to more appropriate strategies. The results of some oral diseases are considered to be acceptable provided they fit within the context of the person. For example, teeth tend to darken as a person ages. Within this definition it would be considered appropriate for the person, but in our first suggested definition of oral health (based on WHO 1946) it might be considered a change that needed reversal.

Health care consumes huge resources. How do we know whether people are healthier as a result of this spending on health care? Deciding whether health has improved is complex and requires a definition and appropriate measure of health in order that goals may be set and achieved by a strategy. But it is also important that 'what health care decision makers achieve should be what is valued most highly by those who benefit and those who must pay' (Sheill 1995). There is an imperative, therefore, to close the gap between the definition of need as perceived by the provider and that perceived by the consumer of health care (Cushing *et al.* 1986).

DISCUSSION POINTS

At what point does a malocclusion become a health problem?

CONCLUSION

This chapter has discussed the definition of health in general and of oral health in particular. Although it appears to be relatively straightforward, it can be seen that the definition of health is more complex than was first thought. It is determined by a complex interplay of many factors: experiences, cultural identity, and socio-economic status. As a result it is important not to make assumptions about any individual's or group's views and it is necessary to avoid stereotyping. An erroneous definition of health can lead to inappropriate use of resources.

REFERENCES

Blaxter, M. (1990). *Health and lifestyles*. London, Tavistock.

Bowling, A. (1997) *Research methods in health: investigating health and health services.* Buckingham, Open University Press.

Bradshaw, J. (1972). A taxonomy of social need. In *Problems and progress in medical care*, 7th series (ed. G. McLachlan), pp. 69–82. Oxford University Press.

Carr, W. and Wolfe, S. (1979). Unmet needs as a socio-medical indicator. In *Sociomedical health indicators* (ed. J. Ellision and A. E. Siegman), pp. 33–46. Farmingdale, Baywood.

Cooper M. H. (1975). *Rationing Health Care*, London, Croom Helm.

Culyer, A. (1976). *Need and the National Health Service: economic and social choice*. London, Martin Robertson.

Cushing, A., Sheiham, A., and Maizels, J. (1986). Developing socio-dental indicators: the social impact of dental disease. *Community Dental Health*, **3**, 3–17.

Dolan, T. (1993). Identification of appropriate outcomes for an aging population. *Special Care in Dentistry*, **13**, 35–9.

Ewles, L. and Simnett, I. (1999) *Promoting health: a practical guide to health education.* London, Baillière Tindall.

Hart, N. (1985). *Themes and perspectives in sociology: the sociology of health and medicine.* Ormskirk Lancashire, Causeway Press.

Herzlich, C. (1973). *Health and illness*. London, Academic Press.

James M. (1999) Towards an integrated needs and outcome framework. *Health Policy* **46**, 165–77

Locker, D. (1988). Measuring oral health: a conceptual framework. *Community Dental Health*, **5**, 3–18.

Naidoo, J. and Wills, J. (1996). *Health Promotion: foundations for practice*. London, Baillière Tindall.

O'Mullane, D., and Robinson, M. (1977). The distribution of dentists and the uptake of dental treatment by school children in England. *Community Dentistry Oral Epidemiology*, **5**, 156–9.

Reisine, S. (1985). Dental health and public policy: the social impact of dental disease. *American Journal of Public Health*, **75**, 27–30.

Scrambler, G. (1997). Health and Illness behaviour. In *Sociology as applied to medicine*, 4th edn (ed. G. Scrambler), pp. 35–46. London, Saunders.

Sheiham, A. and Spencer, A. (1997). Health needs assessment. In *Community oral health* (ed. C. M. Pine), pp. 39–54. London, Wright.

Sheill, A. (1995). Health outcomes are about choices and values: an economic perspective on the health outcome movement. *Health and Social Care*, **3**, 105–14.

Tudor Hart, J. (1971) The inverse care law. *The Lancet*, **Vol. I**, 405–12.

WHO (World Health Organization) (1946). *Constitution*. Geneva, WHO.

WHO (World Health Organization) (1984). *Health promotion: a discussion document on the concept and principles*. Copenhagen, WHO.

Zola, I. (1972). Pathways to the doctor: from person to patient. *Social Science and Medicine*, **7**, 677–89.

FURTHER READING

Locker, D. (1988). Measuring oral health: a conceptual framework. *Community Dental Health*, **5**, 3–18.

Naidoo, J. and Wills. J. (1996). *Health promotion: foundations for practice*. London, Baillière Tindall.

Scrambler, G. (1997). Health and Illness behaviour. In *Sociology as applied to medicine*, 4th edn (ed. G. Scrambler), pp. 35–46. London, Saunders.

4 Public health approaches to prevention

CONTENTS

By the end of this chapter you should be able to:

- Describe differing strategy approaches in prevention.
- Outline the stages necessary in planning any strategy.
- Describe the rationale for choosing between approaches.
- Outline the principles of screening.
- Design a strategy to tackle a major oral health problem.

This chapter links with:
- Definitions of health (Chapter 2).
- Overview of epidemiology (Chapter 5).
- Trends in oral health (Chapter 6).
- All chapters in Part 3 (Chapters 9–16).

INTRODUCTION

Oral diseases are preventable and are very common. What is going wrong? Why have these diseases not been prevented? The answer to these questions is not straightforward. As highlighted in Chapter 2, a complex array of factors influence the health status of individuals and populations. Many of these factors are outside the control of health professionals and the health services. If oral diseases are to be prevented, it is necessary to have a strategy or a plan to tackle the determinants. This chapter discusses the principles of strategy design with reference to prevention. Firstly, it considers the basic principles that need to be addressed when preparing any strategy. Secondly, it examines the various approaches that can be taken when considering prevention and discusses the advantages and disadvantages of each. It looks at issues concerning selection of population groups and individuals through screening, and considerations involved in designing a strategy to tackle a major oral health problem.

PRINCIPLES OF STRATEGY DESIGN

The existence of a strategy implies that there is an organized plan to reach a goal. In this sense designing preventive strategies is similar to other health care planning. The same elements must be present (Box 4.1).

It is important to have a clear vision of what you are trying to achieve and how it is planned to get there otherwise it is unlikely that the goal will ever

> **Box 4.1** Principles of strategy design
>
> **Aim:**   What is to be achieved?
> **Objectives:**   What are the steps that eventually mean this aim is reached?
> **Data collection:** Identify the problem.
>   Understand the problem.
>   Possible solutions.
>   Evaluation and feedback into strategy design.

be realized. The first stage is to identify the aim of the project. What is to be achieved? The second stage is to identify the objectives of the project. What are the various steps that will eventually mean that the aim is reached?

To formulate the aims and objectives of a programme it is necessary to collect data to provide information. Asking a series of questions can facilitate this. These data will include the following.

Identifying the problem

What is the problem that is to be addressed? Is it, for example, caries in pre-school children or early identification of oral cancer?

Understanding the problem

What is the natural history of the disease? What are its aetiology, risk factors, and predisposing factors? What is its epidemiology? Is the incidence increasing, decreasing, or stable? How important is the disease within the population? It may be important in two ways: it may affect many people within the population or it may affect few people but be of major impact.

Understanding the possible solutions

What effective interventions are there? What is the scientific basis for believing that the intervention is effective? What are the means of delivering these interventions? How do these interventions link with other conditions? Will they increase or reduce other conditions? What resources are required? Who else is interested/disinterested in the problem under consideration? Who might help/hinder the implementation of the strategy?

DISCUSSION POINTS

In planning a preventive strategy it is necessary to identify the resources that would be required to implement that strategy. What is meant by the term resources? What does it include and what should it include?

Understanding the evaluation phase

Evaluation should not only include whether the aim was achieved but also whether the objectives were achieved. The factors that helped and hindered the implementation should be recorded. Evaluation is not something that is done at the end of a project but should be built into it. Evaluation should ask questions such as: Does it work? Is it acceptable to people? Is it reaching the people that it is meant to reach? How are the resources being used? Is the resource utilization appropriate? What is the public health perspective on the proposed strategy? Evaluation should be fed back into the design phase of the strategy so that the strategy is constantly updated and monitored and the lessons of implementation are incorporated into any new design.

The planning cycle is a useful review of the necessary stages in developing a strategy (Fig. 4.1). It should be a continuous process, so that when the first evaluation is completed the problem is reassessed, and the question 'Is it time to stop?' is constantly asked.

RISK

Attempting to prevent a disease is only worthwhile if there is a risk of that condition occurring. Immunization programmes for smallpox were practised until the 1970s, when the disease was eradicated from the world. The risk of now contracting that disease is almost zero and there is no need to continue the immunization programme. This example is at one end of the spectrum, but most conditions and risk factors are far more difficult to make judgements about. Preventive strategies are about reducing risk by altering the determinants of disease. How those determinants affect the rate at which disease occurs in the population has an effect on the approach that is adopted towards preventing that disease. The rate is not necessarily constant (Rose 1992).

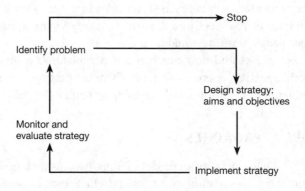

Fig. 4.1 The planning cycle.

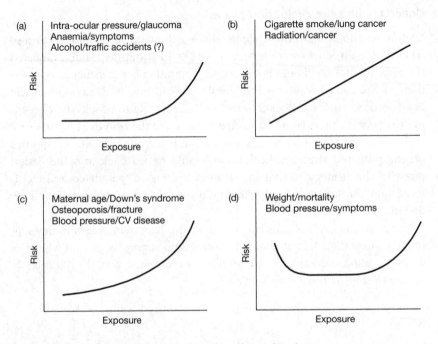

(a) | Intra-ocular pressure/glaucoma
Anaemia/symptoms
Alcohol/traffic accidents (?)

(b) | Cigarette smoke/lung cancer
Radiation/cancer

(c) | Maternal age/Down's syndrome
Osteoporosis/fracture
Blood pressure/CV disease

(d) | Weight/mortality
Blood pressure/symptoms

Fig. 4.2 Schematic models of four possible relationships between exposure to a cause and the associated risk of disease. (Reproduced from Rose 1992 with permission. See Permissions.)

Rose (1992) presented four possible relationships between exposure to a cause and the associated risk of disease (Fig. 4.2), each of which will need different approaches to prevention. Example (b) shows the relationship between cigarette smoking and lung cancer. In this situation any reduction in exposure is likely to be accompanied by a reduction in disease. Choosing an approach that reaches the whole population is appropriate. Example (c) shows a scenario where significant risk is likely to occur mainly at greater levels of exposure, and an approach that reaches only those at high risk may be preferable. Example (a) is a case where there is no increase in risk until a particular level is reached, while example (d) shows increasing risk at both ends of the spectrum, illustrating a case where it may be desirable to move people towards a middle point.

The concept of risk and how much risk is acceptable is of major importance in deciding which approach to take. There is rarely no risk, so in altering determinants to health it is only possible to reduce the risk.

STRATEGY APPROACHES

Rose (1992) divides strategy approaches into two distinct groups: those aimed at the whole population and those in which certain sections of the population are identified, either as a group or as individuals. The first approach is known as the whole-population approach, and the second as the risk approach. The risk approach has two subdivisions. Where population subgroups are identified it is known as the directed or targeted approach, and where individuals are identified it is known as the high-risk approach.

The whole-population approach

If a disease is normally distributed in the population then everyone has some disease. Assuming that the decision is made to try to reduce the overall disease burden, the choice is between trying to reduce everybody's exposure to the agents that are responsible for the disease or to select a subgroup of the population at the right-hand end of the distribution, those at highest risk. Rose is strongly in favour of the whole-population approach in this case. He considers that risk factors affect all who live in society and it is therefore more effective to work with the whole population (Fig. 4.3). Rose posed the fundamental question: does a small increase in risk in a large number of individuals generate more cases than a large increase in risk in a few individuals?

Another justification of the whole-population approach is when the results of not intervening to prevent a condition in even one person are very severe. The outcome in that person may be devastating or the costs to society of not treating that condition may be very great.

One often-quoted problem (Box 4.2) is that sometimes, although it is known that the whole population would benefit, there just may not be enough money or personnel to provide the intervention. This is more usually a problem with clinically based interventions than with environmental change programmes. It then means that hard decisions have to be made. Batchelor (1998) argued that more dental caries might be prevented by con-

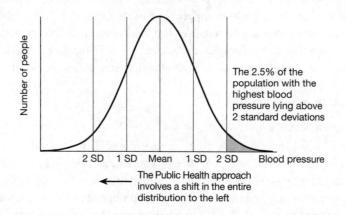

Fig. 4.3 A hypothetical normal distribution of a disease within a population. (Reproduced from Ashton and Seymour 1988 with permission. See Permissions.)

Box 4.2 Strengths and limitations of the whole-population approach

Strengths

Radical   A whole-population approach that seeks to remove the underlying impediments by addressing the social and political factors confronts the root causes and is radical.

Powerful   A small shift in the population distribution of the risk factors may have a large effect on the number of people affected.

Appropriate   Changing the normal behaviour of the population to accepted behaviour for good health.

Limitations

Acceptability   Although a particular change may be obvious it may not be acceptable to the population and they may not be willing to make personal changes or support environmental changes.

Feasibility   Other pressures within society may make the changes very hard to bring about.

Costs and safety   The costs have to be paid immediately but the benefits are more long term. Reducing access to risk factors may adversely affect some people. Rose gives the example of the social disruption to long-term residents when bad housing is demolished.

(Adapted from Rose 1992.)

---

centrating on a whole-population approach, as more caries will occur in those with low levels of disease.

Examples of a whole-population approach

Water fluoridation is an excellent example. Dental caries is one which affects most people and the strategy is to alter the environment by adjusting the level of fluoride in the water supply. The advantages are that everyone on the centralized water supply receives the intervention so that compliance is not a problem. Other examples include seat belt legislation, where all car passengers are required to wear seatbelts, and smoke-free environments.

The risk approach

The targeted-population approach

This works on the principle that some groups of the population are at greater risk compared with the whole population (Fig. 4.4). A variety of interventions can be used: it may be a clinical intervention, more of an environmental approach, or the developing of community and individual skills. It is important to note that this approach means that not all people who are at risk of the disease will be included within the target group. It may be a useful approach particularly where resources are limited or where one

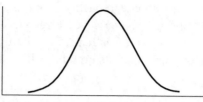

Hypothetical normal distribution of disease in the
population

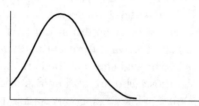

Hypothetical distribution of disease after successful
application of the whole-population approach

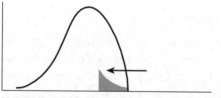

Hypothetical distribution of disease after successful
application of the high-risk approach

Fig. 4.4 A comparison of the effects of the whole-population and high-risk
approaches.

group is clearly more disadvantaged than another. With the emphasis on
reducing inequities in health this approach is more in favour. It differs from
the high-risk approach in that not every person within the targeted group
is at higher risk but as a whole the group is. With the high-risk approach
every person targeted is at increased risk.

Examples of a targeted-population approach

Identifying a section of the population as being at greater risk of dental
caries may lead to the decision to provide a targeted-population approach.
An example of this might be a small geographical area that has been
found to have much higher levels of dental decay. The schools are identified and a decision is made to introduce a fluoride toothpaste brushing
scheme.

In Cardiff a targeted-population approach is being used to try to improve the health of people living in an area called Riverside. All the housing in this area is being refurbished, and it is hoped that by upgrading the environment of this targeted population, its overall health will also improve.

The High-risk approach

The high-risk approach is used when the treatment of only those at greatest risk is considered most appropriate. Rather than using the whole population or part of it, only specific individuals are identified by a screening programme. Before deciding that a high-risk approach is what is required, consider the advantages and disadvantages (Box 4.3). It is only of benefit if it can identify those in the population who are at most risk of developing a condition and if there is an effective way of preventing that condition. It will inevitably miss some people who will contract the condition of interest. By definition 'high risk' omits those who are at 'low risk', but 'low risk' does not mean 'no risk'. This may or may not be acceptable to either decision makers or the public. If a screening test is used then the specificity and sensitivity must be of an acceptable level. These terms are defined below, but to summarize: high values of these ensure that people with a high risk will be identified and those without will not.

Examples of a high-risk approach

Dental students are required to demonstrate their hepatitis status before entering the dental course. There are two reasons for this. Firstly, to ensure the public's safety by not letting infected people undertake invasive proce-

---

Box 4.3 Strengths and weaknesses of the high-risk approach

Strengths
- Intervention is appropriate to the individual.
- It avoids interference with those who are not at special risk.
- It is readily accommodated within the ethos and organization of medical care.
- It offers a cost-effective use of resources.
- Selectivity improves the benefit-to-risk ratio.

Weaknesses
- Prevention becomes medicalized.
- Success is only palliative and temporary.
- The strategy is behaviourally inadequate.
- It is limited by a poor ability to predict the future of individuals.
- There are problems of feasibility and cost.
- The contribution to overall control of a disease may be disappointingly small.

(Modified from Rose 1992.)

dures, but secondly, to enable an effective immunization to be administered as part of the strategy to stop the dental students contracting a potentially fatal illness. In the UK this high-risk approach is satisfactory, only immunizing those who are most at risk (by virtue of their occupation). In other countries where the disease is endemic a whole-population approach is more likely to be appropriate.

Another condition where a high-risk approach is taken is in suggesting to all women who have lost a close relative to breast cancer before the age of 50 that they have regular mammograms. Mammograms have not been shown to be effective in the whole population in this age group but it is of use in those with a higher risk of contracting the disease. They are limited to women over the age of 50 where effectiveness has been shown.

Finally, in people who have received irradiation of their salivary glands it is highly appropriate to provide a very intensive programme of clinical prevention because of their known greatly increased risk of developing dental caries.

DISCUSSION POINTS

Which approach would you take to dealing with pre-school caries in a population with high caries? Would this be any different if there was a high prevalence of the disease in the population compared with a low prevalence?

PRINCIPLES OF SCREENING

Screening has been defined as:

> The presumptive identification of unrecognized disease or defect by the application of tests, examinations or other procedures which can be applied rapidly. (Commission on Chronic Illness 1957)

In the context of prevention the aims of screening are:
• To protect society from contagious disease.
• To identify people who are at high risk of a disease either for preventive or early treatment interventions.
Holland and Stewart (1990) described four types of screening. These are:
• Screening for individuals with risk factors which predispose to disease but are not themselves alerting symptoms.
• Screening for individuals with early signs of disease.
• Screening for individuals for which preventive action could be taken to restore health.
• Screening for established disease that could be alleviated by continuous care and surveillance.

Compared with clinical diagnosis screening is cheap and rapid, but less accurate.

When people are screened one of four results may arise. They are:

- **True positive** The test was positive and the individual did have the disease.
- **False positive** The test was positive and the individual did not have the disease.
- **False negative** The test was negative and the individual did have the disease.
- **True negative** The test was negative and the individual did not have the disease.

Four statistics are used to describe the results of a screening test. They are:

- **Sensitivity** The probability of a positive result if the disease is present.
- **Specificity** The probability of a negative result if the disease is absent.
- **Positive predictive value** The probability that the disease is present if the test is positive.
- **Negative predictive value** The probability that the disease is absent if the test is negative.

The first two of these measures relate purely to the validity and reliability of the screening test, while the last two also include a measure of the disease prevalence. In broad terms a high positive predictive value is dependent upon a high prevalence in the population. The closer the sensitivity and specificity are to one the closer is the screening test to achieving 100% accuracy. This is very rarely achieved and as a result some positive cases may be missed and some negative cases may be referred for further investigation.

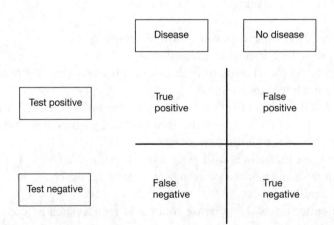

Fig. 4.5 Sensitivity and specificity.

In assessing the value of a screening test, its acceptability and cost also need
to be considered. Further, it is essential that there is some benefit to having the
screening test. There is little point in identifying a person as having a condition if there is nothing that can be done to improve their situation.

There are problems arising from screening programmes. The first is that
if the screening programme is ineffective it may result in inappropriate use
of resources. It may lead to over-diagnosis which may result in the treatment of trivial conditions. Screening may lead to misdiagnosis. If a false
negative result is given it may elicit false reassurance, and even encourage
a person to ignore other symptoms that they should act upon. Finally, the
amount of fear and anxiety that screening tests cause should not be
underestimated.

Wilson and Jounger (1968) described ten principles of screening:
1. The condition should be an important health problem.
2. There should be an accepted treatment for patients with recognized
   disease.
3. Facilities for diagnosis and treatment should be available.
4. There should be a recognizable latent or early symptomatic stage.
5. There should be a suitable test or examination.
6. The test should be acceptable to the population.
7. The natural history of the disease, including its development from
   latent to declared disease, should be adequately understood.
8. There should be an agreed policy on whom to treat as patients.
9. The cost of case-finding (including diagnosis and treatment of patients
   diagnosed) should be economically balanced in relation to possible
   expenditure on medical care as a whole.
10. Case finding should be a continuous process and not a 'once and for all'
    project.

PREVENTION FOR INDIVIDUALS

In dentistry there are several clinically effective preventive techniques available, for example fissure sealants and professionally applied fluorides. Where do these techniques fit into a preventive strategy? It is important to understand that individual prevention is really another form of treatment. As such it has many of the problems associated with traditional operative care. The preventive techniques may be aimed at a specific subgroup of the population but if those people have problems accessing dental care or they experience other barriers to dentistry, then it is unlikely that they will be able to receive these preventive techniques. Individually based prevention requires compliance. Unless alternative methods of delivery are used it is highly probable that the desired level of uptake will not be achieved. The inverse care law can be as applicable to preventive care as to treatment. Offering preventive care without a strategy may even increase health inequalities because it can often be those who least need the prevention who take it up. All the limitations of the medical model approach also apply to prevention for an individual. It can thus be seen that trying to use individual prevention with a section of the population requires an innovative approach.

Over the years attempts have been made to use fluoride-rinsing programmes in schools with varying amounts of success. Above all else, the use of individual methods of prevention does not use the common risk-factor approach and does little to alter the determinants of disease which are, after all, the factors that caused the problems. It also is important that any individual method is subject to evaluation and monitoring. It may be that the problem fluoride-rinsing was introduced to solve no longer exists or is being prevented in an alternative way. A good example of this was a school fluoride mouth-rinsing programme in the United States. Over time the prevalence of dental caries in the population dropped, the cost–benefit of using a mouth-rinse became much smaller, and the total benefit to the population was greatly reduced. It was thus decided that the most sensible course of action would be to cease the programme. However, this proved much more difficult than had been anticipated (Disney *et al.* 1990).

Before selecting a preventive technique it is important to examine it in the same way as one would a treatment option. A series of questions need to be

DISCUSSION POINT

Imagine a young single mother with two pre-school children living on social security benefits and based some 3 miles from the nearest health centre. It is recommended to her that she should attend the local dentist on several occasions to have her elder child's first permanent molars sealed. Discuss the benefits and limitations of recommending this care to this family.

asked. Is the technique effective? Is it accessible to the desired target population? Is it acceptable to those people? Is it affordable to whoever is responsible for paying? Preventive techniques should also be clinically effective.

PREVENTION FOR POPULATIONS

Population prevention can adopt many different ideas. However, excluding those items which are really individual methods, for example immunization, the preventive techniques that are most useful are those that focus on the determinants of health. By following the principles of the Ottawa Charter (see Chapter 9) it is possible to bring about change that does not require action by individuals to ensure compliance and success.

In Chapters 1 and 9 the common risk-factor approach to disease is outlined. By working across several diseases using the common risk-factor approach, it is likely that this will have more success than other approaches that are limited to one disease. It also makes better use of the limited resources that are available and thus better economic sense.

Smoking is an excellent example: the use of multiple approaches has led to a fall in the rates of smoking in the UK. Clearly the most relevant factor is the ensuing drop in the rates of lung cancer but this reduction in smoking may also be implicated in the lower levels of periodontal disease that are now recorded. What are these multiple approaches? Firstly, there have been education campaigns. There have been changes to the legislation surrounding the advertising and sale of tobacco. The range of tobacco products available for sale is less than in other parts of the world; for example, it is not possible to buy products designed for chewing. The environment has been altered by creating 'no smoking' zones. Today it is hard to imagine that half of all double-decker buses used to be thick with smoke and that it was not possible to eat in a non-smoking area of a restaurant. As well as these environmental and legislative changes, emphasis has been placed on teaching general medical practitioners and other health care staff to instruct and support people who wish to give up smoking. Finally, in acknowledgement of the fact that nicotine is a very addictive substance, nicotine patches have been introduced which allow people to withdraw from it. Initially these were only available by purchasing them but they are now also available on prescription. Making the patches available on prescription is a very simple way of improving access for those with less income. Otherwise the advent of patches might well have led to an increase in inequalities.

It is important to realise that results are not instant. It may take many years to bring about dramatic changes in the smoking rates of the population. However, there is evidence that rates of smoking and rates of smoking-related cancers are declining. It is more difficult to relate these changes to the interventions described above.

DISCUSSION POINT

The use of alcohol in the UK is similarly subject to considerable environmental and legislative control. Using the Ottawa Charter (Chapter 9) for the major domains, identify factors that are in place to try to reduce alcohol-related problems.

The evaluation of population-based prevention is particularly difficult to undertake, especially measuring its success by examining changing patterns of disease. However, other types of evaluation are easier. The success of the process can be examined, investigating how many people participated in a screening programme or what has happened to cigarette sales following a health education campaign.

DISCUSSION POINT

Refer again to the example of the single mother given on p. 58. How might population-based measures and the common risk-factor approach be used in this case?

OTHER CLASSIFICATIONS OF PREVENTION

A very commonly described classification of prevention defines preventive levels as primary, secondary, or tertiary. Although this is often seen, it is now considered out of date and has been superseded by the methods described above. It is described here for completeness and also to explain why it has been replaced. This is most easily done by example, using dental caries.

Primary prevention Dietary control or use of fluoride toothpaste to prevent the start of the carious process.

Secondary prevention Use of fluoride to arrest an early carious lesion or fissure sealant to arrest an occlusal lesion.

Tertiary prevention Restoration of the tooth to restore form and function and to arrest the carious lesion.

As the example shows, the classification concentrates more on the disease process and the individual rather than the aetiological or risk factors and the population. It is also, as Ewles and Simnett (1999) point out, difficult to distinguish when one type of prevention stops and the next stage starts.

CONCLUSION

A preventive strategy needs to be based upon a good needs assessment of the problem, an evaluation of the interventions available, and careful consideration of the most appropriate method for delivering the desired intervention. This must include an assessment of which population, part of the population, or individuals need to be included. Prevention delivered to individuals is liable to encounter all the problems of treatment services and alternative delivery methods may be needed to avoid these. A whole-population strategy is best if it adopts multiple approaches using legislative, environmental, and individual interventions. It is possible that a preventive strategy will increase inequalities if this specific aspect is not addressed.

REFERENCES

Ashton, J. and Seymour, H. (1988). *The new public health*. Milton Keynes, Open University Press.

Batchelor, P. (1998). The scientific basis for the modelling of caries preventive strategies. PhD Thesis, University of London.

Commission on Chronic Illness (1957). *Chronic illness in the United States*. Commonwealth Fund, Cambridge, Mass, Harvard University Press.

Disney, J., Bohannan H., Klein, A., *et al*. (1990). A case study in contesting the conventional wisdom: school-based fluoride mouthrinse programs in the USA. *Community Dentistry and Oral Epidemiology*, **18**, 46–54.

Ewles, L. and Simnett, I. (1999). *Promoting health: a practical guide*. London, Baillière Tindall.

Holland, W. W. and Stewart, S. (1990). *Screening in health care*. London Nuffield Provincial Hospitals Trust.

Rose, G. (1992). *The strategy of preventive medicine*. Oxford, Oxford University Press.

Wilson, J. and Jounger, G. (1968). *The principles and practice of screening for disease*. Geneva, WHO.

FURTHER READING

Murray, J. (ed.) (1996). *The prevention of dental disease* (3rd edn). Oxford, Oxford University Press.

Pine, C. (ed.) (1997). *Community oral health*. Oxford, Wright.

Rose, G. (1992). *The strategy of preventive medicine*. Oxford, Oxford University Press.

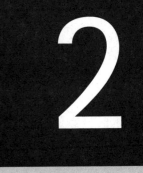

2

Oral epidemiology

5 Overview of epidemiology

CONTENTS

By the end of this chapter you should be able to:

- Define epidemiology and its requirements.
- Describe the uses of epidemiology.
- Outline the steps necessary to undertake an epidemiological study.
- Understand the different types of epidemiological study and how they apply to dental care.
- Understand the principles of measuring dental disease.
- Be able to describe the ideal features of an index and know some of the limitations of existing indices.

This chapter links with:
- Trends in oral health (Chapter 6).
- Prevention and oral health promotion (Part 3).
- Health economics (Chapter 22).
- Public health approaches to prevention (Chapter 4).
- Evidence-based dentistry (Chapter 7).

INTRODUCTION

How tall is the human race? What is meant by being short? Walking down the street one will see people of various heights and a degree of variation exists. Some people are shorter than others but when is someone abnormally so? How is it possible to make this judgement?

By recording the height of everyone it is possible to start to produce a picture of people as a whole. Such terms as minimum, maximum, and mean give an indication of the distribution of heights. The science used to collect and examine data in this way is known as epidemiology. Epidemiology is defined as:

The orderly study of diseases and conditions where the group and not the individual is the unit of interest (Mausner and Kramer 1985).

Mausner and Kramer (1985) state that epidemiology is concerned with the frequencies of illnesses and injuries in groups of people as well as the factors that influence their distribution. By investigating differences between subgroups of the population and their exposure to certain factors it is possible to identify causal factors and consequently to develop programmes to alleviate the problems. The critical issue is that knowledge is gained by studying patterns in groups as opposed to concentrating solely on the individual.

This chapter gives an overview of the uses of epidemiology in dentistry and describes the main principles of this subject.

Epidemiology in dentistry operates in two broad fields. These are:

1. The measurement of dental disease among groups within the population in order to understand factors that influence the distribution, and
2. Evaluation of effectiveness of new materials and treatment in clinical trials and assessment of needs and requirements for dental services within the community.

DISCUSSION POINTS

Why is it important to know if different sections of the community have different disease patterns?

Undertaking epidemiological investigations requires a series of standards and procedures; measures must be made to an agreed common standard, in a methodological manner and, when necessary, using an appropriate random sample. For example, taking again the example of height, using a basketball team or a kindergarten class as a sample would give misleading data as to the inferred heights of the population in general. These examples give an indication of some of the issues that must be considered in epidemiology. This chapter will describe some of these issues with particular relevance to dentistry.

HOW EPIDEMIOLOGY IS DIFFERENT

Epidemiology is the scientific method of studying diseases in populations. It is different from both clinical examination and from screening. The differences are outlined in Table 5.1.

Epidemiological studies: the protocol

All epidemiological investigations require a protocol that follows scientific method. The aim of writing a protocol is to describe in great detail the thinking behind the proposed study and the exact methodology. This chapter describes the process of designing a study and is complemented by the chapter on critical appraisal which looks at the process of appraising a paper. Some examples of protocols have been published (Palmer *et al.* 1984;

Table 5.1 Comparison of clinical diagnosis and epidemiology and screening

Epidemiologist	Screening	Clinical practice
Applied to populations or samples of selected groups	Offered to selected groups or individuals	Offered to individual who present at a practice
Criteria relate to the purpose of the study	The identification criteria are related to the need for follow-up	Diagnosis aims to form the basis for treatment
Findings inform subsequent action	Follow-up offered to those identified as needing it	Treatment is provided

Box 5.1 Purposes of a protocol

- To ensure the study is well thought through and adequately planned.
- To allow the study to be evaluated for scientific and ethical factors prior to starting.
- To ensure that the investigators complete the study as planned.
- To allow others to complete the study for the original investigator, if necessary.
- To enable others to repeat the study.

Pine *et al*, 1997a, b; Pitts *et al.* 1997; WHO 1997) and are useful as a basis for writing further studies.

Background

What previous work has been done in the general area? What has been learned? What mistakes have been made? What was done well? What was done badly? By answering these questions it should be possible to formulate questions that can become aims and objectives.

Aims and objectives

The aims of a study are the questions that are being answered while the objectives are the steps it is necessary to go through to answer the questions. The aims are extremely important. They should be clear and, most importantly, should not attempt to answer too much.

In descriptive studies, aims and objectives are often sufficient. However, in analytical studies it is usually necessary to also formulate a hypothesis. For example, in a clinical trial that has the aim of comparing the caries-preventive effectiveness of two toothpastes:

The *objectives* would be to measure and compare the caries increment in two groups of children aged, say, 12 years, over a given time period, say 36 months.

The *hypothesis* would be that there is a difference in caries preventive effectiveness between the two toothpastes.

The *null hypothesis* would be that there is no difference in caries preventive effectiveness between the two toothpastes. The null hypothesis is used because it is impossible to prove something, one can only disprove an accepted hypothesis. Statistical tests are used to identify the chance of the observed results occurring.

Study design and sampling

The first important point is to choose an appropriate study type. The second important point is to decide upon the population that would be appropriate for the study and to consider whether and how a sample should be drawn.

Sometimes it may be appropriate to include the whole population within the study but more usually a subgroup is selected. The key principle of sampling is that it must be representative of the population from which it is drawn. This is achieved by randomly sampling all the people in the eligible group in such a way that every individual has an equal chance of being selected. Analyses based upon a random sample can then be used to describe the population with appropriate statistical limitations being placed upon the interpretation. A random sample should be used wherever possible.

Imagine the situation where it is necessary to achieve a random sample of 5-year-old children from schools. A simple way is to sample in stages. First to sample schools, and then children within the schools. This is called 'stratification'. It may be necessary to weight schools to ensure that all children still have an equal chance of being selected (Pine *et al.* 1997).

Other forms of research use samples such as the 'quota' sample. In essence this means identifying people who meet predetermined criteria and asking them to participate. This method is used in market research and also in some qualitative research. The problem with this type of sampling is that there may be some characteristics in common between the people who are prepared to take part in the research that influence the results. It is important to acknowledge that this may be so when the data are being analysed.

The sample size for any study is critical. A statistician should be consulted to ensure that sufficient subjects are included for any proposed study where comparisons are to be made. If too few people are selected then it is possible that a real difference which exists may not be identified. Overall costs may increase for no real benefit if too many subjects are used.

Data collection

The aims, choice of study design, and the selected population or sample will provide information on both the type of data and the frequency with which they need to be collected. In the example above where two toothpastes are to be compared in a clinical trial, it can be seen that data have to be

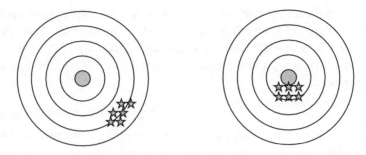

Fig. 5.1 The difference between reliability and validity.

gathered on at least two occasions (baseline and end of study) on two groups (one for each toothpaste).

It is necessary to decide what is to be measured. In the example of the toothpaste a clinical examination will be required to evaluate the caries status. However, it might be considered that extra information would be gained by taking bitewing radiographs or that the acceptability of the toothpaste to the clients needed to be measured by a questionnaire or interview.

A principle aim of data collection is to ensure that valid, reliable, and unbiased data are collected. Valid means that the data measure something that truly exists accurately. Reliable means that if measurements are taken on a different occasion the same answer is obtained. Unbiased means that neither the subject nor the examiner influences the finding (see Fig 5.1).

Is it possible to construct the study so that it is blind or double blind? Blind means that the subject is not aware whether they are in the test or the control group and double blind means neither the subject nor the assessor is aware. With trials such as toothpaste it is relatively easy to hide which group an individual is in, but if a trial is comparing an amalgam restoration with a composite restoration this is not possible.

Training and calibration of the examiners and recorders in the measures and criteria to be used is necessary. It is important to keep *inter-examiner* variability (variation between different examiners) and *intra-examiner* variability (variation within examiners) to a minimum. This is achieved through training and calibration and monitored by re-examining a percentage of subjects or administering questionnaires on a second occasion to measure the reproducibility.

Prior to starting the main study, a pilot study should be undertaken to check all stages of the proposed study using the predetermined criteria. Any modifications can then be made.

A standard system for recording data needs to be agreed and training given as errors are surprisingly common.

Analyse data

It is very important to plan the data analysis **before** the start of the study. As with estimating the sample size, a statistician should be consulted to assist in the planning. This serves two purposes: the investigator needs to explain the types of data being collected and the reasons for doing so; the statistician can advise on the correct analyses and any limitations. If a pilot study has been completed the data from that should be analysed to see if problems exist.

Draw conclusions

The conclusions of the study are the only part that cannot be described in detail in the protocol because they are not known. They should relate back to the aims and objectives and not to other matters. For example, in the previous example of the toothpaste study it would be unacceptable to conclude that, as there was no difference between the toothpastes, a programme of fissure sealants should be implemented. The study had never set out to evaluate fissure sealants.

Dissemination

The final stage of a study is dissemination. Even if only negative results were found it is important that these are communicated to the scientific community.

Ethical approval

This is required for any study involving the collection of data on human subjects. In all areas of the country there are Local Research Ethical Committees (LRECs). The ethics committee, which must be contacted before commencing a study, will ensure that the study is scientifically sound and ethical. The committees are composed of medical researchers and lay people. Lay representation is very important in ensuring the project's acceptability to the potential subjects.

Box 5.2 Factors examined by an ethics committee

- Satisfactory scientific design.
- That the information given to the subject is adequate and comprehensible.
- That the proposed subjects are competent to give consent.
- That the consent is voluntary.
- That the risks and benefits of participating in study are fully explained.
- That issues of confidentiality and data protection are adequately handled.

DISCUSSION POINTS

Why is it important to have ethical approval? What might be the problems to the subjects and to the investigators of not having it?

TYPES OF STUDY

Descriptive epidemiology

Descriptive epidemiology, as its name suggests, describes patterns of disease, risk factors, and determinants of health in a population or subgroup. The data are described in such terms as:

- Who is affected: which age groups, which sex, which ethnic or occupational groups?
- Where does the condition occur: in which countries or population subgroups, and when?

There are two types of descriptive data:

Routinely collected data

Much data are gathered in this way. There is a legal requirement to record all deaths in the UK and the reason for the death is given on the death certificate. The Acheson Inquiry used these data and reported on the social class differences between people (Acheson 1998). More specifically, for oral health, all cases of oral cancer are registered and it is possible to analyse in whom and where cases are occurring. Changes in the incidence of cancer over time can also be identified and variations proven to help start examining why they exist. Examples of research using these data include MacFarlane *et al.* (1993) and Hindle *et al.* (1996).

Cross-sectional studies

These are surveys designed to identify the levels of a condition and associated risk factors at the same time. While easy and rapid to undertake, they are not able to establish cause and effect. For example, if unemployed people are more likely to be ill, if the data are gathered at the same time, it is impossible to identify whether being unemployed makes people ill or whether being ill stops people getting jobs.

Despite the limitations, the method of investigation is much used in dentistry. Regular surveys of the oral health of people are undertaken, some of which are described in Chapter 6. Examples used include O'Brien (1994), Pitts *et al.* (1998, 1999, 2000), and Kelly *et al.* (2001).

Because descriptive surveys cannot be used to establish cause and effect, alternative study designs need to be adopted, namely analytical studies.

Analytical studies

Observational

In epidemiology, inferences can be made from observing what people do or have done in the past. It may not be possible to alter a risk factor experimentally, for example, a study investigating the effects of smoking. It would be unacceptable to involve people in a study in which they were required to start smoking. The effects of smoking are known to be detrimental and the study would not be allowed on ethical grounds. To examine the effects of smoking, a study could only compare people in the population who already smoke with those who do not. As a result, the study always carries the risk of misinterpretation. Some other factor may explain why people who smoke have poorer health.

Observational studies are either retrospective (go back in time) or prospective (go forward in time). In retrospective studies, also known as case-control studies, people with the condition of interest are identified: for prospective studies, also known as cohort or longitudinal studies, people who have a higher exposure to the risk factor than normal are identified. For each type of study, the identified group is matched with controls and the groups monitored in prospective studies or questioned in retrospective studies to describe what risk factors in the past they may have been exposed to. By comparing the incidence of the condition and the exposure rates it is possible to test hypotheses as to what may be causing the condition.

DISCUSSION POINTS

What problems could occur if reliance is placed on people's memories? What other ways exist of gathering retrospective data and what problems may arise?

The findings from the observational studies can be further investigated in experimental studies.

Experimental or interventional
Randomized clinical trials

These are experimental and prospective. They are regarded as the most appropriate mechanism through which causal relationships can be established and described by some as the 'gold standard' of research. They are most useful in the evaluation of new materials and drugs. RCTs are based on the principle that the two groups used are identical in all respects except in the subject of the study. In the simplest design, subjects are randomly allocated to two groups. One group receives the test treatment and the other a placebo. A true placebo (no treatment) is rarely allowed on both ethical grounds and the difficulty in ensuring the study is blind. In consequence, the control group usually receives what is the current best treatment. Ideally the study should be undertaken blind or double blind. Baseline measures are made and the subjects followed over time. Differences in the results of treatment are compared between the two groups to see if the new treatment is superior to the old.

In dentistry, a common variation on this design exists in which the mouth is split down the middle. It is often seen in trials that evaluate dental filling materials; subjects would have to have two similar cavities on the opposite side before entering the trial. The test material can then be compared in the same environment to the control material. A good example of this type of trial is that reported by Welbury *et al.* (1991).

Community trials

These are also experimental and prospective. However, in some instances it is not possible to randomly allocate people to test and control groups, but rather groups of people, for example, schools in a health education pro-gramme. It would be very difficult to stop students discussing the types of health education they had received and therefore the control group does not really exist. It would be impossible to know what type of intervention each student had had. While it is an acceptable design, such studies need to be handled statistically in a different way to normal using cluster analysis as there may be common factors within each group that affect the results.

Natural experiments

Very occasionally an event may occur that gives a possibility of evaluating something that would not otherwise be possible. This is most easily explained using the example of the dropping of the atomic bombs at Hiroshima or Nagasaki. Their use provided an opportunity to study the rela-tionship between the dosage of radiation received, based on how far people lived from the explosion epicentre, and its effect on them. The results pro-vided data that are used to estimate the safety levels of radiation for humans.

DISCUSSION POINTS

What do you think the practical problems of undertaking prospective studies might be?

Systematic reviews

The appropriateness of including systematic reviews here centres on their value as a method for assessing the quality of the literature covering a topic. In situations where a number of clinical trials addressing the same question have not been consistent, an overview of the trials, a systematic review, can be made using the statistical technique of meta-analysis. The technique pools the results of the studies to gain an estimate of the over-all effect from the combined clinical trials. There are a number of impor-tant requirements that the summary data from the clinical trials need to comply with and when considering undertaking such a study expert statistical advice is essential.

CAUSATION AND ASSOCIATION

In the previous section, the relevance of each study design in helping to identify causality was noted. While two factors may occur together, this does not
imply that the presence of one leads to the other. The relationship may simply be associative. For example, suppose it was found that people who travel
by aircraft are more likely to develop skin cancer. Is the mode of travel the
causative factor or was it purely an association? The more plausible explanation is that people who travel by aircraft are more likely to sunbathe for
longer. To reach the beach to sunbathe they travelled by aeroplane. The
causal factor is far more likely to be exposure to the sun than aircraft travel.
    Mausner and Kramer (1985) describe the commonly used criteria, often
referred to as Bradford Hill's criteria (see Box 5.3), to judge whether the relationship between two factors is causal or just an association.

MEASURING HEALTH

To be able to make comparisons between the health of different groups or
in the same group at different times, it is necessary to measure a condition.
More often than not this is achieved by measuring an illness or disease
rather than health itself.

Box 5.3 Bradford Hill's criteria

Strength of the association: the ratio is calculated for the disease rates for those
with and without the causative factor. The greater the ratio the more likely it is to
be a causal relationship.

Dose–response related: increasing amount of the causative factor would lead to
increasing amounts of disease.

Consistency of the association: that the finding is similar in different places, in
different populations, and with different study methods.

Correct with respect to time: exposure to the causative factor must occur before the
disease develops and should also allow for any latent period.

Specificity of the association: this criterion suggests that every time the causative
factor occurs there will be a case of the disease. The closer to a one-to-one
relationship the greater the specificity. A one-to-one relationship is very rare,
occurring in some types of cancers, and this criterion is less important than the
preceding ones.

Biological plausibility: there should be biological plausibility for the supposed
causative factor.

Reversibility: if the causative factor is removed there should be less cases of the
disease.

(Adapted from Mausner and Kramer 1985.)

Rates

A rate is a measure of how disease progresses over time. The most commonly used rates are the death or mortality rate in a population, either in general or for a given condition, and the illness or morbidity rate.

Mortality rates

Mortality rates are measured by collecting information from death certificates. A death certificate contains considerable information, including the individual's name and date of birth, along with the primary and, if appropriate, secondary causes of death. The cause of death is, however, only as accurate as the diagnostic ability of the person completing the form.

DISCUSSION POINTS

Certain conditions may be under-reported on a death certificate. The most common of these are murder and suicide. Give some reasons why this might be so?
What would be the public health implications of this under-reporting?

Directly comparing mortality rates can be very misleading without taking a variety of factors into consideration. For example, suppose one population has a higher death rate from cancer compared to another. The first population may be significantly older and thus would be expected to have a higher cancer death rate. To establish whether the difference is due to a particular causative agent or simply natural factors, a method of controlling for factors known to be related is required. This is addressed by standardizing factors such as age and presenting standardised mortality rates (SMRs). These enable true comparison of mortality rates.

Morbidity rates

Morbidity rates are much more difficult to calculate accurately for the majority of diseases and conditions. Certain disease, primarily infections, have to be notified. These include measles, meningitis, and tuberculosis. It is possible to get a fairly good idea of how many cases of these diseases are being identified by doctors but not possible to know how many remain undiagnosed in the community.

How much of a specific disease is there in a given population? This can be very difficult to ascertain as on many occasions it is answered only by analysis of routinely collected data. For example, how could one establish how many people in the population have lower back pain? Surrogate data may be collected by establishing absentee rates from work, or by attendance at the doctor, but neither of these methods comes close to identifying all the people in a population who may have lower back pain, let alone the severity of the condition. The other problem is that it cannot be presumed that people will report back pain at a similar point in their history. Some groups of the population may not visit a doctor at all and continue working while the condition may interfere much more with other people's lives, causing them to seek help at a much earlier point. Using routinely collected data may give a biased assessment of the true picture. Often the only way to collect reliable and complete morbidity data is to undertake a specific survey where the diagnostic criteria are explicit and agreed.

In dentistry specific surveys are performed to examine the dental health of the population. In the UK there are two major groups of surveys. The first is the decennial surveys of Adult and Child Dental Health, and the second are the BASCD (British Association for the Study of Community Dentistry) co-ordinated surveys. These use random samples of the population, agreed criteria, and trained and calibrated examiners. They are cross-sectional surveys and describe the oral health of their study populations at one point in time. They are also useful for examining changes over time in the health of the population; see the section covering trends in oral health.

DISCUSSION POINTS

In the UK specific surveys of oral health are performed to examine the dental health of the population. These use random samples of the population, agreed criteria, and trained and calibrated examiners. What are the advantages of this assessment of oral health? What are the disadvantages?

Prevalence and incidence

Prevalence

Prevalence is the percentage of a population that have the disease in question now, divided by the population at risk.

For example, the prevalence of influenza in a population of dental students would be the number of students who have influenza now divided by the total number of dental students. For prostate cancer the population at risk would exclude women.

Incidence

Incidence is the number of new cases of a disease divided by the population at risk in a given time period.

The incidence of influenza in a population of dental students would be the number of new cases of influenza divided by the total population of dental students over a time period, usually of a year.

The word incidence is used differently in trials investigating dental caries. Rather than using the person as the unit for describing a new case, the tooth or even the surface is used. The incidence of dental caries is therefore expressed as the increase in DMFT or DMFS scores (see p. 81 for an explanation of DMFT and DMFS) over two points in time. It is better termed the 'increment'.

WHY INDICES ARE USED

At its most simple, an index is an instrument that enables the quantity of a disease or a state to be measured. In dental epidemiology indices are developed in order to measure diseases, for instance dental caries, tooth erosion, or gum disease.

For example, in order to evaluate a new fluoride toothpaste, agreement by those making the assessment on what constitutes decay in a tooth is required. If the examiners are unable to demonstrate that they can diagnose to a similar standard, then any variation between groups may be related to the variation between the examiners rather than to the effects of the new toothpaste. To help address this and other potential problems, an agreed set of criteria and the conditions under which they are applied are necessary.

Such measures are called indices. Standardization takes place at the beginning of a study and may also be made at various points throughout its course to ensure that there is no alteration in the diagnostic criteria being used. It is important that standards remain the same within the same examiner at different times (intra-examiner variability) and between different examiners at the same time (inter-examiner variability). Statistical tests are used to measure the amount of variability.

The development of indices allows comparisons between different studies and between different data sets. However, when there have been no training exercises between the investigators any comparisons must always be treated with a degree of caution due to the possibility of a change in diagnostic standards. The great advantage of indices is that, despite their limitations, trends may be identified which are useful in helping define what subsequent investigations need to be undertaken.

Properties of an ideal index

The properties of an ideal index are related to the index's purpose. An index is there to measure change within groups and differences between groups. The purpose of the index is to act as a measuring system that reduces the amount of invalid variation. An index that will come closest to achieving this should have a number of properties. See Box 5.4.

Examples of dental indices

Most commonly used dental indices measure disease rather than health. They measure biological changes and examples are listed in Table 5.2. Most of the examples are categorical in nature.

Box 5.4 Properties of an ideal index

Simple

The index should be easy to understand and easy to learn how to use. This is important as if it is not, invalid measurement variation is likely to arise.

Objective

The index should be objective to use. It should not be susceptible to the examiner's opinion. The categories should be clear-cut so that it is easy to make a decision as to which category a condition should fit into. The index should also relate to the clinical stages of the condition it is measuring.

Valid

The index must measure what it intends to measure. If the index is measuring dental caries it must measure dental caries and not, for example, enamel hypoplasia. The index should also bear a relationship to any 'gold standard' for diagnosing the condition. When a positive finding is found by the index it should also be found by the gold standard and vice versa. In statistical terms it should have good sensitivity and specificity.

Reliable

Each time the index is used it should find the same result. This is different to the next category, 'reproducible', as reliability is concerned with the internal workings of the index not the variation caused by examiners. In other words there should not be variation on occasions of use as a result of an internal flaw within the index.

Reproducible

The index must give the same result if the condition being assessed has not changed. This must be true if it is the same examiner measuring at different times or a different examiner measuring the condition at the same or a different time. These issues apply equally if it is the subject who is undertaking the measurements, for example by completing a questionnaire.

Quantifiable

The index should provide a measurement on which statistical analyses can be undertaken, for example it might calculate the mean and distribution of the data collected. Many indices use categorical measurement scales of a condition; for example, a male, female, or oral hygiene index that uses good, fair, and poor. It is important to distinguish whether an index is numerical or categorical, as producing mean figures for, say, data collected on the CPITN index is wrong.

Sensitive

The index should be able to detect small changes. Ideally, an index should be able to measure change in either direction, that is, whether the condition being measured improves or deteriorates, although certain conditions are irreversible; for example, a DMF score.

Acceptable

Any index, when being applied to a subject, should be acceptable. It should not be painful, or embarrass or demean them. The length of time to complete any assessment should also be borne in mind.

Table 5.2 Commonly used dental indices

Index	Use	Reference
DMFT/dmft	Measurement of caries	Klein *et al.* 1938
CPITN (BPE)	Periodontal treatment need	Ainamo *et al.* 1982
	Plaque	Loe and Silness 1963
	Gingivitis	Silness and Loe 1964
DDE modified	Enamel defects	Clarkson and O'Mullane 1989
TF index	Fluorosis	Thylstrup and Fejerskov 1978
Dean's index	Fluorosis	Dean 1934
Horowitz index	Fluorosis	Horowitz 1986
IOTN and PAR	Orthodontic treatment need and assessment of treatment need	Shaw *et al.* 1991
Trauma index	Trauma	O'Brien 1994
Erosion index	Erosion	Walker *et al.* 2000
RCI	Root caries	Katz 1980

BPE: Basic Periodontal Examination
CPITN: Community Periodontal Index of Treatment Need
DDE: Developmental Defects of Enamel
TF: Thyslstrup and Fejerskov
IOTN: Index of Orthodontic Treatment Need
PAR: Peer Assessment Rating
RCI: Root Caries Index

Other indices may simply be a measurement involving length or depth, for example millimetres when assessing pocket depth or loss of attachment.

Measuring dental caries

The DMF/dmf index is commonly used to measure the prevalence and severity of dental caries in a population. The index is used separately for the primary and the permanent dentition. Upper-case letters (DMF) are used for the permanent dentition and lower-case letters (dmf) for the primary dentition. When a count is made of the number of teeth the total is known as the DMFT score. A variation on the index is to use tooth surfaces as the assessment unit as opposed to the tooth. This variation is known as the DMFS or dmfs index.

Decayed due to caries (D or d).
Missing due to caries (M or m).
Filled due to caries (F or f).

> **Box 5.5** Calculating the treatment index, the care index, and the restorative index
>
> The treatment index is $((M + F) / DMF) \times 100$
> The care index is $(F / DMF) \times 100$
> The restorative index is $(F / (D + F)) \times 100$

The components are then totalled to give a DMF score for an individual. Other measures can be calculated using data collected by the DMF index; for example, the proportion of the disease that has been treated can be calculated. Three measures can be used: the treatment index, the care index, and the restorative index. Box 5.5 illustrates how they may be calculated. These measures are helpful in giving some indication of which sections of a population are getting treatment and what types of treatment they are receiving.

The DMFT index is an historical index; it records not only current disease but also previous disease. Some problems with the index are summarized in Box 5.6. How do we ensure that a missing tooth has been lost due to decay and not for some other reason? How do we decide whether or not a tooth is decayed? While this may vary from study to study, for nationally collected data in the UK the criteria are standardized through training programmes.

DISCUSSION POINTS

What other reasons are there for teeth to be missing from the mouth besides caries?
What might be the implications for reporting the number of missing teeth (MT) in a sample of 15-year-olds?

Measuring periodontal disease

Accurate measurement of periodontal disease is much more difficult, not least due to the lack of what constitutes periodontal disease. In recent years, the index most commonly adopted has been the Community Periodontal Index of Treatment Need (CPITN) (Ainamo *et al.* 1982), but as its name describes this is an assessment of treatment need, not of the amount or the activity of periodontal disease. Within the general dental service this index has been adapted and re-named the Basic Periodontal Examination (BPE), where it is used to identify those patients in need of a more detailed periodontal examination. In this instance it is used as a screening test. The CPITN is useful for describing the prevalence of need for different types of treatment but it is not suitable for measuring the effectiveness of treatments. In this instance it is far more useful to use specific clinical indicators such

---

Box 5.6 Problems with the DMF index

Relevance

The relevance of DMF to caries experience assumes that missing and filled teeth were once carious. Teeth may be missing for other reasons such as trauma or periodontal disease.

Treatment decisions

A restoration may be placed for preventive reasons (e.g. preventive resin restoration of a tooth with an early lesion) rather than restorative reasons (e.g. amalgam restoration for restoring a carious tooth). The DMF cannot distinguish between the two and the level of caries experience may be inflated.

Quality of teeth

The DMF assigns equal weight to filled, missing, and decayed teeth. An individual with 10 decayed teeth or 10 missing teeth will score the same as one with 10 filled teeth. The implications for their dental health may be different but the index does not make any distinction.

Benefit of treatment

Filled teeth score the same as missing teeth, implying that there is no difference and no benefit to having decayed teeth restored.

Irreversible

The DMF index is irreversible: an individual's total score can only increase over time. Consequently it is of limited value when assessing whether there have been improvements in an individual's health.

(Sheiham et al. *1987)*

---

as presence or absence of bleeding or the loss of attachment to measure disease progression.

Limitations of existing indices

While indices have continued to change and develop, knowledge of the natural history of disease has also changed. For example, the traditional view of periodontal disease as a series of progressions from mild gingivitis to severe periodontal disease has been discounted. The limitations of the DMF index have been discussed previously. Perhaps more fundamentally, the indices continue to measure disease as opposed to health. Various researchers, for example, for DMF data Sheiham *et al.* (1987) and Marcenes and Sheiham (1993), have tried to tackle this problem by analysing the data gathered in different ways. The first proposal (F-health) was termed a functional measure of health and gave equal weight to filled and sound teeth and zero weighting to decayed teeth. The second proposal was the T-health where proportional weights were given to sound, filled, and decayed teeth. This later modification conceptual-

---

Box 5.7 The functional health and tissue health indices

F-health (FH) = Sound Teeth + Filled Teeth
T-health (TH) = (Sound Teeth x 4) + (Filled Teeth × 2) + (Decayed Teeth × 1)

(Marcenes and Sheiham 1993)

---

izes sound teeth as best, filled teeth as good but not as good as sound, and decayed teeth as having the possibility of restoration as they have not been extracted. These composite measures of dental health status attempt to give a better indication of the function and quality of the dentition.

The newer indices

Bowling (1991) outlines the problems facing people who are trying to measure health. She points out that, particularly for chronic diseases, measuring disease rates is now no longer sufficient. It is far more important to describe the social and psychological effects of the problem, as well as the more traditional aspects, on the quality of life.

DISCUSSION POINTS

In what ways can oral ill health limit or interfere with day-to-day life?

Existing indicators of oral disease fail to measure the impact of disease, impairment, and health care on people's well-being; they are professionally based and do not take account of people's perception of need. The biomedical model of disease predominates.

Locker (1988) argued for a conceptual model of oral health which defined health not only as an absence of disease but also included functional aspects along with social and psychological well-being. The model focuses on optimal functioning and social roles, thus addressing many of the limitations of normative clinical need assessment. It has provided the context for the development of oral health-related quality of life measures (OHQoL) which are described in Chapter 21. Locker's conceptual model is reproduced in Fig. 5.2. For a more detailed discussion of the model and its relationship to need see Chapters 3 and 21.

This diagram suggests that, if disease works in this way, the measurement of changes in discomfort or functional limitation, rather than disease, would be more appropriate for assessing the effects of ill health and intervention. The degree of handicap may be a better measure than disease. Think again about the difference between a filled front tooth and a missing front tooth. Both of these score 1 on the DMFT index but do they both affect a person's life in the same way? Do they both affect everybody's lives in the same way?

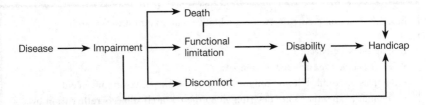

Fig. 5.2 The conceptual model of health, adapted from WHO 1980. (Reproduced from Locker 1988 with permission. See Permissions.)

DISCUSSION POINTS

At what point does a malocclusion become a health problem? Similarly, what treatment should be provided for gingivitis?

While it is difficult to measure how conditions such as these affect individuals, doing so gives some distinct advantages. For example, in the debate about what treatments are provided, priorities can be set for those conditions that affected or impacted on people's lives more. Alternatively, an index for comparing the effectiveness of treatments, not in terms of clinical outcomes but in terms of improvement to the quality of life of the person, might be developed.

Such measures are far more complex and difficult to develop. Examples are in use for both general health and, more specifically, oral health. A detailed description is outside the scope of this book but the two oral health examples are those defined by Slade and Spencer (1994) and Leao and Sheiham (1996).

Questionnaires

These are a common way of collecting data. However, they require considerable skill in construction. The principles of data collection apply equally when developing questionnaires. Where possible it is sensible to use questionnaires that have been developed and tested for a similar study. Questionnaires are limited in general to the current state of knowledge on a topic. They also tend to reflect the researchers' view of key issues. Questionnaires have the advantage that data on large numbers of people can be collected, but they may lack depth. In addition, transferring questionnaires either into different cultures or languages is not straightforward; the wording may mean something very different in one situation when compared to another. This is why piloting is so important. Furthermore, people sometimes complete questionnaires in a way that reflects well upon themselves rather than what they really think or do.

> **Box 5.8** Main differences between qualitative and quantitative research
>
> In qualitative research:
> • Fewer people are included in samples.
> • Samples are unlikely to be random but may be purposive or convenient.
> • The matters discussed are determined by the research subjects rather than by the researcher.
> • Greater quantities of more detailed data are collected.

Qualitative research

Epidemiology has concentrated on quantitative methods. However, not all data can be gathered using quantitative methodologies nor analysed using the more conventional methods. An alternative method that address the shortcomings is qualitative methodology.

Qualitative techniques obtain data through two main sources: the focus group and the one-to-one interview. These may be structured, with the investigators having a list of topics that they want the subjects to discuss. Alternatively they may be semi-structured where, although there are some topics to be discussed, the interviewers want the lead the subjects through the interview in a particular manner. A third alternative is when the interviews are totally unstructured. The interviewer's role is to facilitate the process and not to contribute to it.

Irrespective of the method adopted, it is very important for the interviewer to be independent so as not to bias the findings. The interviews are often tape-recorded or very detailed notes are made. This second method is less desirable. The interview tapes are transcribed and can either be analysed by hand or by using a software package such as NUD*IST. The purpose of the analysis is to identify themes that arise in several of the interviews. Once identified, the researcher attempts to create structured data by categorizing responses into patterns.

Qualitative data may be used in a variety of different ways. They may be used to develop questionnaires for subsequent quantitative testing. Data can also be used for reporting themes or ideas to inform policy and decision-making. Less often they are used after quantitative research to try to add detail or reasons to the results.

CONCLUSION

Epidemiology is the study of disease and risk factors in groups. The study methodology, sampling, and measuring tools are important aspects in this science. With the development of evidence-based dentistry there is an increasing need to understand the principles of epidemiology.

REFERENCES

Acheson, S. D. C. (1998). *Independent Inquiry into Inequalities in Health Report*. London, The Stationery Office.

Ainamo, J., Barmes, D., Beagrie, G. *et al.* (1982). Development of the World Health Organization (WHO) community periodontal index of treatment needs (CPITN). *International Dental Journal*, **32**(3), 281–91.

Bowling, A. (1991). *Measuring health: a review of quality of life measurement*. Milton Keynes, Open University Press.

Clarkson, J. and O'Mullane, D. (1989). A modified DDE Index for use in epidemiological studies of enamel defects. *Journal of Dental Research*, **68**, 445–50.

Dean, H. T. (1934). Classification of mottled enamel diagnosis. *Journal of the American Dental Association*, 1424–6.

Elderton, R. and Nuttall, N. (1983). Variation amongst dentists in planning treatment. *British Dental Journal*, **154**, 201–6.

Hindle, I., Downer, M. C., Speight, P. M. (1996). The epidemiology of oral cancer. *British Journal of Oral and Maxillofacial Surgery*, **34**(5), 471–6.

Horowitz, H. S. (1986). Indexes for measuring dental fluorosis. *Journal of Public Health Dentistry*, **46**, 179–83.

Katz, R. V. (1980). Assessing root caries in populations: the evolution of the root caries index. *Journal of Public Health Dentistry*, **40**(1), 7–16.

Kelly, M., Steele, J., Nultall, N. *et al.* (2001). *Adult Dental Health Survey: oral health in the United Kingdom, 1998*. London, The Stationery Office.

Klein, R., Palmer, C., Knutson, J. W. *et al.* (1938). Studies on dental caries 1. Dental status and dental needs of elementary school children. *Public Health Report (Washington)*, **53**, 751–65.

Leao, A. and Sheiham, A. (1996). The development of a socio-dental measure of dental impacts on daily living. *Community Dental Health*, **13**, 22–6.

Locker, D. (1988). Measuring oral health: a conceptual framework. *Community Dental Health*, **5**, 3–18.

Loe, H. and Silness, J. (1963). Periodontal disease in pregnancy. I Prevalence and Severity. *Acta Odontological Scandinavia*, **21**, 533–51.

MacFarlane, G. J., Evstifeeva, T. V., Scully, C., *et al.* (1993). The descriptive epidemiology of pharyngeal cancer in Scotland. *European Journal of Epidemiology*, **9**(6), 587–90.

Marcenes, W. S. and Sheiham, A. (1993). Composite indicators of dental health: functioning teeth and the number of sound-equivalent teeth (T-Health). *Community Dentistry and Oral Epidemiology*, **21**(6), 374–8.

Mausner, J. and Kramer, S. (1985). *Epidemiology, an introductory text*. Philadelphia, Saunders.

O'Brien, M. (1994). *Children's dental health in the United Kingdom 1993*. London, HMSO.

Palmer, J. D., Anderson, R. J., Downer, M. C. (1984). Guidelines for prevalence studies of dental caries. *Community Dental Health*, **1**(1), 55–66.

Pine, C. M., Pitts, N. B., Nugent, Z. J. (1997a). British Association for the Study of Community Dentistry (BASCD) guidance on sampling for surveys of child dental health. A BASCD coordinated dental epidemiology programme quality standard. *Community Dental Health*, **14** (Suppl. 1), 10–17.

Pine, C. M., Pitts, N. B., Nugent, Z. J. (1997b). British Association for the Study of Community Dentistry (BASCD) guidance on the statistical aspects of training and calibration of examiners for surveys of child dental health. A BASCD coordinated dental epidemiology programme quality standard. *Community Dental Health*, **14** (Suppl. 1), 18–29.

Pitts, N. B., Evans, D. J., Pine, C. M. (1997). British Association for the Study of Community Dentistry (BASCD) diagnostic criteria for caries prevalence surveys – 1996/97. *Community Dental Health*, 14 (Suppl. 1), 6–9.

Pitts, N. B., Evans, D. J., Nugent, Z. J. (1998). The dental caries experience of 12-year-old children in the United Kingdom. Surveys coordinated by the British Association for the Study of Community Dentistry in 1996/97. *Community Dental Health*, **15**(1), 49–54.

Pitts, N. B., Evans, D. J., Nugent, Z. J. (1999). The dental caries experience of 5-year-old children in the United Kingdom. Surveys co-ordinated by the British Association for the Study of Community Dentistry in 1997/98. *Community Dental Health*, **16**(1), 50–6.

Pitts, N. B., Evans, D. J., Nugent, Z. J. (2000). The dental caries experience of 14-year-old children in the United Kingdom. Surveys coordinated by the British Association for the Study of Community Dentistry in 1998/99. *Community Dental Health*, **17**(1), 48–53.

Shaw, W. C., Richmond, S., O'Brien, K. D., *et al.* (1991). Quality control in orthodontics: indices of treatment need and treatment standards. *British Dental Journal*, **170**(3), 107–12.

Sheiham, A., Maizels, J., Maizels, A. (1987). New composite indicators of dental health. *Community Dental Health*, **4**(4), 407–14.

Silness, J. and Loe, H. (1964). Periodontal disease in pregnancy. II Correlation between oral hygiene and periodontal condition. *Acta Odontological Scandinavia*, **22**, 120–35.

Slade, G., Strauss, R., Atchison, K., *et al.* (1997). Measuring oral health and quality of life. Chapel Hill. University of North Carolina, Dental Ecology.

Slade, G. D. and Spencer, A. J. (1994). Development and evaluation of the oral health impact profile. *Community Dental Health*, **11**, 3–11.

Thylstrup, A. and Fejerskov, O. (1978). Clinical appearance of dental fluorosis in permanent teeth in relation to histologic changes. *Community Dentistry and Oral Epidemiology*, **6**, 315–28.

Walker, A., Gregory, J., Bradnock, G. *et al.* (2000). *National Diet and Nutrition Survey: young people aged 4 to 18 years*. London, The Stationery Office.

Welbury, R. R., Walls, A. W., Murray, J. J. (1991). The 5-year results of a clinical trial comparing a glass polyalkenoate (ionomer) cement restoration with an amalgam restoration [see comments]. *British Dental Journal*, **170**(5), 177–81.

WHO (World Health Organization) (1997). *Oral health surveys: basic methods*. WHO, Geneva.

FURTHER READING

Babbie, E. (1990). Survey research methods (2nd edn). Wadsworth, Belmont, California.

Babbie, E. (1992) The practice of social research (6th edn). Wadsworth, Belmont, California.

Bloor, M., Frankland J., Thomas, M., and Robson, K. (2001). *Focus groups in social research*. Sage, London.

Mays, C. and Pope, N. (1999). *Qualitative research in health care*. BMJ Publications, London.

Mausner, J. and Kramer, S. (1985). *Epidemiology, an introductory text*. Saunders, Philadelphia.

6 Trends in oral health

CONTENTS

INTRODUCTION

In the introduction to Chapter 1 it was stressed that in order to decide whether a disease is a public health problem it is important to be able to answer some key questions about it. Is the disease widespread? Is it on the increase? What individuals or groups appear to be susceptible? Do we know what causes it? Can it be prevented? What is the impact of the disease on the individual and society? The epidemiology of oral diseases can provide some detailed answers to these important questions. This chapter will present a brief overview of trends in oral diseases for children and adults in the UK. It will focus on periodontal disease, oral cancer, and dental caries but there is a brief section on dental trauma and erosion. Dentofacial anomalies, per se, are not diseases, but will be included here, as their prevalence and incidence have implications for dental care because of the impact on social and psychological well-being. The problems of oral health inequality will be reviewed and the implications of trends in oral diseases for dental care in the UK will be discussed.

There are many surveys describing the oral health of children and adults in the UK, with decennial national surveys of both groups since 1973. In these surveys all dental examiners are trained and calibrated, so that the diagnostic criteria are consistent and national trends can be identified. See Chapter 5 for a brief description of the importance of standardization of diagnostic criteria. In addition the British Association for the Study of Community Dentistry (BASCD) undertakes surveys of the oral health of children within the districts of the UK; again, examiners are trained and calibrated and changes in trends in oral health across Health districts and regions can be monitored at shorter intervals than in the 10-yearly national surveys.

PERIODONTAL DISEASE

Epidemiology

Current concepts in relation to periodontal disease have changed considerably in the last 20 to 30 years. The traditional 'progressive' disease model has been replaced by the 'burst theory'. That is, periodontal diseases have short 'bursts' of activity followed by long periods of remission and healing (Goodson *et al.* 1982; Socransky *et al.* 1984). While gingivitis is widespread, it does not inevitably lead to premature tooth loss. For the majority of the population periodontal disease progression is slow (Pilot 1997). Only 5% of the population experience destructive periodontal disease and this is declining (Burt 1988). The severity and rate of destructive periodontal disease does not lead to significant tooth loss or pain and discomfort in the majority of populations. See Chapter 14 for a more detailed account.

Young people rarely experience severe destructive periodontal disease. The National Diet and Nutritional Survey 2000 reported on the periodontal health of children aged 4 to 18 years (Gregory *et al.* 2000). Within this age range 35% were recorded as having unhealthy gums, with the proportion increasing with age. Gingivitis occurred in 40% of 15–18-year-olds, as evidenced by bleeding; 17% of this group had pocketing with boys twice as likely to be affected as girls. Two-thirds of the children aged 4 to 18 years reported that they brushed their teeth at least twice per day and 8% less than once per day. The younger children (4–6 years) and older children (15–18) were more likely to brush their teeth. Girls were more likely than boys to brush their teeth.

In the UK, 54% of adults had some periodontal pocketing of 4 mm or more and 5% had severe pocketing (greater than 6 mm) (Kelly *et al.* 2000). Attachment loss and prevalence of pocketing increased with age: 43% had attachment loss of less than 4 mm and 8% had attachment loss of greater than 8 mm. Nearly three-quarters of dentate adults had visible plaque on their teeth and 73% had some calculus. The frequency of tooth-brushing was associated with presence of visible plaque: those who reported brushing their teeth at least twice per day had less visible plaque than those who brushed their teeth at least once per day or never. The frequency of tooth-brushing did not appear to have an impact on periodontal disease (Nunn *et al.* 2001).

A survey of older people living in the community and in institutions found that around 22% had periodontal pockets of 6 mm or more, with an average of 2.3 teeth affected (Steele *et al.* 1998). Oral and denture hygiene were poor, and worse in the institutionalized group.

Aetiology

Many factors have been associated with periodontal disease, but dental plaque is the most important. Others include smoking, certain systemic diseases, stressful life events, and local factors (poor restoration contour) contributing to plaque accumulation. Calculus (tartar) does not itself lead to periodontal disease (Jenkins 1996). It does, however, promote plaque retention. Periodontal diseases occur rarely in children.

Treatment

Frandsen (1986) carried out a review of treatment interventions for periodontal disease. He cast doubts on the effectiveness of common periodontal treatments such as scale and polishes, removal of calculus, and root planing. In the absence of a sound evidence base for the treatment of periodontal disease, the best strategy is to focus on prevention through tooth-cleaning, refraining from smoking, and minimizing local factors in the mouth which may contribute to plaque accumulation.

Implications for the future of trends in periodontal disease

The changing concepts of periodontal disease and the associated difficulty in developing predictors of periodontal disease mean that judgements about future treatments are difficult. However, gross destructive periodontal disease is experienced by a small group of people (about 5%) and it would appear to be declining. The treatment options are poorly evidence-based. The best option would appear to be in developing public health strategies to promote oral cleanliness and reduce smoking. Oral hygiene remains a problem for UK adults with 75% having visible plaque on their teeth (Nunn *et al.* 2001).

DISCUSSION POINTS

Are periodontal diseases a public health problem? Use the example of adolescents to illustrate your answer.
Why do you think adolescent boys do not brush their teeth as often as girls?
How would you convince a young male teenager to brush his teeth more frequently?

ORAL CANCER

Epidemiology

Oral cancer is usually taken to include cancer of the lip, tongue, gingiva, floor of the mouth, and other unspecified parts of the mouth. In the UK there are about 2000 new cases and 900 deaths from oral cancer annually. The disease is twice as common in men as women. Incidence increases with age and 85% of cases are found in those aged 50 and above (Cancer Research Campaign 2000).

Trends

Between 1911 and the early 1970s there was a steep decline in mortality for male oral cancers (Cancer Research Campaign 2000). There are indications that the incidence and mortality rates have begun to increase again, particularly in young men and women (Boyle *et al.* 1993). The reasons for this are unclear. As survival rates after treatment are not good, the best option for management of oral cancer is to invest in prevention through reduction in alcohol and tobacco use.

Aetiology

The causes of oral cancer are well documented, and are divided into established risk factors and predisposing factors. The two most important risk factors (accounting for 75–90% of all cases) are tobacco and alcohol use (Cancer Research Campaign 2000). Dietary deficiencies in vitamins A, C, E, and iron are known predisposing factors. The changing incidence is thought to be due to altered alcohol use but this has not been confirmed.

Treatment

While progress has been made in the treatment of oral cancers, survival rates have not improved (Stell and McCormick 1985). The 5-year survival rate is 50%, but this does increase to 80% when there is early detection (Cancer Research Campaign 2000). See Chapter 15 for a more detailed account of screening, trends, and prevention.

Implications for the future of trends in oral cancer

It would appear that the incidence and mortality rates for oral cancers are on the increase. The best strategy for the future would appear to lie in early detection of oral cancers and health promotion activities aimed at reducing the consumption of alcohol and tobacco products.

DENTAL CARIES

Epidemiology

There have been dramatic changes in the pattern and distribution of dental caries in children and adults in the UK over the last 25 years. The epidemiology of dental caries in the UK will be briefly described for pre-school children and 5-year-olds, children with a permanent dentition, adults, and older people.

In pre-school children and 5-year-olds

The National Diet and Nutritional Survey in 1995 found that 40% of toddlers from manual social classes had caries compared to 16% from non-manual classes (Hinds and Gregory 1995). Oral health was worse in Scotland and the north of England. The survey showed that children who commenced oral hygiene practices early had less decay experience than those who started later.

The biggest changes in decay experience were seen in 5-year-olds between 1973 and 1983, when the percentage who were caries free had almost doubled and the dmft had halved (Murray and Pitts 1997). The improvement from 1983 to 1993 is less marked and in the early 1990s evidence from BASCD suggested that the declines in caries experience in 5-year-olds had 'bottomed out' (Palmer and Pitts 1994). However, recent data from BASCD suggest that the overall trend in this group seems 'to be a modest improvement following a long plateau' (Pitts *et al.* 1999). While there are overall declines in dental caries in children in the UK, the regional inequalities in dental health remain (Downer 1994).

The overall number of treated teeth remains low in 5-year-olds. The UK mean care index (f/dmft 100%) is 14% but ranges from 9 to 23% across regions (Pitts *et al.* 1999).

In children with a permanent dentition

The 1993 survey of children's dental health demonstrated the continued declines in dental caries which were seen in 1983 and 1973 (Downer 1994). However, there continued to be wide variation across the UK. At age 8, for example, 62% of English children are caries-free compared to 32% in Northern Ireland (Downer 1994). At age 14, 27% of children in England had active decay compared to 42% in Scotland and 41% in Northern

Ireland (O'Brien 1994). The DMFT for 12-year-olds in the UK was 1.4, which compares well with the WHO DMFT global goal (2000) of 3.0 for industrialized countries.

Dental caries in older groups, 12- and 15-year-olds, continued to decline between 1973, 1983, and 1993. The numbers of caries-free children have increased. Murray and Pitts (1997) suggest that treatment of active decay in certain areas of the UK has been declining. In Scotland, for example, the care index for 14-year-olds (filled teeth as a proportion of total DMF) has fallen from 73% in 1991 to 52% in 1995 (Pitts *et al.* 1995a).

Adult dental health

Steady and substantial improvements in adult dental health were seen in the 1988 national survey compared with the previous national surveys (Downer 1991). The proportion of adults with some natural teeth rose from 70% in 1978 to 79% in 1988 and 87% in 1998, and is expected to reach 90% by the year 2008. It is predicted that 90% of the working-age population should be substantially dentate with 21 or more standing teeth on average by that time (Downer 1991). Younger adults had the most dramatic improvement: there was a sharp increase in the proportion with no restored teeth (otherwise sound) from 9% in 1978 to 13% in 1988 and 30% in 1998. The position for older adults reflected the patterns of disease and treatment experience in earlier times. Northern Ireland, Scotland, and the north of England remained the parts of the UK with the poorest dental health (Downer 1991). The bulk of filled teeth is now found in older adults. Anterior tooth-wear was found to affect 11% of adults (Nunn *et al.* 2001).

Dental caries experience in older people

Edentulousness has decreased in all UK adults since 1968, when 37% of the population over 16 had no teeth (Gray *et al.* 1970). In 1998 edentulousness had declined to 13% (Kelly *et al.* 2000). There was a social class gradient in the experience of edentulousness, with more adults in non-skilled manual households experiencing total tooth loss. In older people the levels of edentulousness are much higher but appear to be declining.

Many older people are retaining part of their natural dentition into later life. For older adults '20 functional teeth' in an acceptable occlusion, free from unsightly gaps and without a need for a partial denture, is a more realistic goal than 32 standing teeth (Kayser 1981; Murray and Pitts 1997). The improvement in adults with '20 functional teeth' was very marked between 1978 (73%) and 1988 (81%) (Murray and Pitts 1997) and 1998 (83%) (Kelly *et al.* 2000). But this goal also considers that the teeth should be in a functional occlusion and without gaps. Table 6.2 shows an analysis of people in 1993 with 21 or more remaining teeth.

When the data are re-analysed to look at the functional and aesthetic elements of dentate people in older life, a different picture emerges. For

Table 6.1 Proportions, past and projected, of adults with 21 or more standing teeth by age, rate of change within cohorts

	1988 Dentate adults with 21 or more standing teeth (%)	1978 Adults with 21 or more standing teeth (%)	1988 Adults with 21 or more standing teeth (%)	1978–88 Rate of change within cohorts (%)	1998 Adults with 21 or more standing teeth (%)	2008 Adults with 21 or more standing teeth (%)	2018 Adults with 21 or more standing teeth (%)
16–24	100	97	100		100	100	100
25–34	96	85	95	−2	98	98	98
35–44	86	65	83	−2	93	96	96
45–54	72	34	60	−5	78	88	91
55–64	48		30		56	74	84
16–64	86		77		87	92	95

Reproduced with permission from Downer 1991. See Permissions.

Table 6.2 Total decay experience of 5-year-old (dmft) and 8-, 12-, and 14-year-old children (DMFT) in England and Wales in 1973, 1983, and 1993 (weighted means), with proportions caries-free

	5 years		8 years		12 years		14 years	
Year	dmft mean	Caries-free (%)	DMFT mean	Caries-free (%)	DMFT mean	Caries-free (%)	DMFT mean	Caries-free (%)
1973	4.0	28	1.7	35	4.8	7	7.4	4
1983	1.8	51	0.7	65	2.9	21	4.7	12
1993	1.8	51	0.3	83	1.2	50	1.9	41

Reproduced from Downer 1994 with permission. See Permissions.

example in 1988, of the 23% of adults over 65 who do retain 20 teeth only, 3% were free from gaps and only 2% had four good quadrants (Murray and Pitts 1997). There is therefore a long way to go for people to attain a functional dentition for life (Murray and Pitts 1997).

Root caries

As people retain their teeth for longer into old age, root caries may become a problem. The extent and nature of the problem is not fully understood as root caries data were only gathered on adults in 1988. In 1998 decay of the root surfaces is uncommon in younger adults (Nunn *et al.* 2001). In those aged over 65 an average of 10.6 teeth were vulnerable and a third had caries. A recent survey of the oral health and diet and nutrition of adults aged 65 and over found that 80% of the roots of the retained teeth had some decay or root restoration (Steele *et al.* 1998). It is possible to overestimate the carious involvement of root surfaces as restored root surfaces are regarded as previously decayed whereas the restoration may have been placed for aesthetic reasons. The Root Caries Index (RCI) (the proportion of vulnerable root surfaces which are unsound) for older people living in the community was 26% compared to 46% for older people living in institutions (Steele *et al.* 1998). Murray and Pitts (1997) suggest that the treatment need for caries in exposed surfaces in older people is now greater than the treatment need for caries in 5-year-olds. Infrequent tooth-brushing and heavy plaque deposits in association with a partial denture were strongly associated with primary root caries in older people (Steele *et al.* 1998).

Aetiology

The cause of dental caries is the consumption of fermentable carbohydrates (sugars). There is a dose–response between the quantity of sugar consumed and the development of dental caries (Sheiham 1991). It is suggested that at levels below 10 kg per person per year (15 kg per person per year in fluoridated areas) dental caries will not develop. It is also known that the greater availability of sugar (Screebny 1983) is associated with increasing dental caries experience in children. Much of these data linking caries and sugar were gathered from retrospective studies. In a prospective survey, Rugg-Gunn (1984) demonstrated that there was a statistically significant difference in caries increment over 2 years in children who were high and low consumers of sugars.

A recent survey of oral health and diet and nutrition in young people (Gregory *et al.* 2000) found that there were links between the frequency of consumption of sugary foods and dental decay. Over half of those examined had evidence of erosion on their teeth.

Treatment

Much of the budget for dental care in the General Dental Service is devoted to the treatment, management, and consequences of dental caries, a disease that has been described as easily preventable (Watt and Sheiham 1999). While there have been substantial declines in dental caries, these have not be linked to the existence of a comprehensive restorative service. The declines in dental caries are attributable to the use of fluoridated toothpastes since their introduction in the middle 1970s (Watt and Sheiham 1999). There has not been any substantial decline in sugar consumption in the UK.

New understanding in relation to the progression of dental caries indicates that there is a potential for an early carious lesion to arrest (Kidd 1996). This means that rather than intervene when early caries is detected, clinicians should opt to monitor the lesion (depending on individual patient factors) and institute preventative measures such as reduction in sugar consumption and local topical application of fluorides (Elderton, 1990). Once the tooth is filled, however small, it enters the 'restorative cycle'. The filling may fail, leak, and require replacement (50% of amalgam fillings had failed 2 years after placement in the General Dental Service in Scotland (Elderton and Davies 1984). The filling will need to be replaced, the cavity will be enlarged, and the potential for failure will increase. Eventually the tooth may need advanced restorative care and ultimately an extraction should that fail. Elderton warns that new understanding of the progression of dental caries demands that the clinical intervention is postponed for as long as possible (Elderton 1996) because lesions have the potential to arrest.

Implications of trends in dental caries

Trends in dental caries indicate that there have been substantial declines in caries experience across all age groups in the last 30 years. In addition, there have been declines in the consequences of dental caries, with many

teenagers and young people having no fillings and the level of edentulousness reducing in older groups. There is, however, a disturbing increase in
oral health inequality, which will be discussed in a later section.

Most experts attribute the declines to the use of fluoridated toothpastes.
Sugar consumption patterns (the cause of caries) have not changed substantially. Fluoridation of the water supplies could bring about further
declines, as could appropriate use of fissure sealants. There is therefore the
potential for further substantial declines, but in the absence of a widespread
dental caries preventive strategy further dramatic declines are unlikely to be
seen.

The pattern and distribution of caries is changing, which has implications
for targeting of resources, dental treatment, and choice of restorative material. In addition, older groups are retaining their teeth for longer and the
incidence and prevalence of root caries may increase. As older people retain
their teeth, there will be a need for more complex restorative treatment, as
they would have entered the 'restorative cycle' in the 1970s and 1980s.
Their dentition may require high maintenance.

The best choice for management of dental caries still lies in its prevention
rather than its treatment. It has been suggested that treatment services
accounted for only 3% of the reduction in dental caries in the 1970s
(Nadanovsky 1995). The established best methods for preventing dental
caries are: reduction in sugar consumption, optimal exposure to fluorides,
and appropriate use of fissure sealants.

TRAUMA

The proportion of children experiencing trauma to their anterior teeth
increases with age from 5% of the 7- to 10-year age group to 18% of the
15- to 18-year group. Boys are almost twice as likely to experience trauma
as girls. The most frequent type of trauma was a fracture in enamel
(Gregory et al. 2000).

EROSION

Dental erosion has been defined as the loss of dental hard tissue by a chemical process that does not involve bacteria. The aetiology of dental erosion
is multifactorial and includes individual anatomy, saliva composition and
flow, intrinsic sources of acid from gastro-oesophageal flux, and consumption of non-milk extrinsic sugars and demineralizing acidic foods (Al-
Dlaigan et al. 2001). Erosion was measured in the 1993 Child Dental Health
Survey and the National Diet and Nutrition Surveys in 1995 (toddlers) and
1998 (4–18-year-olds). The prevalence of erosion was low and increased
with age, 2% of one and a half to two and a half year-olds and 3% of three

and a half to four and a half year-olds had erosion. Erosion is less common in the permanent dentition: 2% of 7-year-olds rising to 12% of 13–15-year-olds had erosion on the buccal surfaces (Hinds and Gregory 1995). On the palatal surfaces it ranged from 7% to 27% in the same age groups. There was little erosion into dentine, ranging from 1% to 2%.

The trends in relation to dental erosion are unclear. The 1998 survey of young people suggested over 50% of children aged 4 to 18 years may have some erosion. It does not appear to be a public health problem at present but many clinicians are reporting a clinical impression that it is increasing (Al-Dlaigan *et al.* 2001). There is a need for careful monitoring as consumption of demineralizing acidic drinks remains high.

DENTOFACIAL ANOMALIES AND ORTHODONTIC TREATMENT NEED

'Malocclusion is not a disease but rather a set of dental variations that have little influence on oral health' (Shaw 1997). Dentofacial anomalies can range from gross disfigurement to minor irregularities in the alignment of the teeth. In the past there was a belief that dentofacial anomalies could compromise oral health but this view is now largely discounted (Shaw 1997). The impacts of dentofacial anomalies are now considered to occur in the social and psychological spheres, in terms of feelings about well-being and appearance. There have been attempts to establish the treatment need in a population and the Index of Orthodontic Treatment Need (IOTN) was developed. It attempts to link the dentofacial variation to perceived aesthetic impairment so that those suffering the greatest impact will be prioritized for treatment (Brook and Shaw 1989).

ORAL HEALTH INEQUALITY

Inequality has been described as health differences which are avoidable, unnecessary, unjust, and unfair (Whitehead 1991). Despite the marked improvement in oral health in children and adults over the last 30 years, there is evidence of widening oral health inequality (Watt and Sheiham 1999).

In children

In children aged 5–15 years, the pattern of attendance is strongly and independently associated with dental decay experience in the primary dentition (Watt and Sheiham 1999). For children aged 12 to 15 years there was an association between class and dental decay. While dental decay declined in all social classes between 1983 and 1993, the gap widened between 12- to 15-year-olds from skilled households (who had improved most) and those from semi-skilled and unskilled households (who had improved least). In 15-year-olds the gap from 1983 to 1993 widened from 0.9 to 1.4 teeth (O'Brien 1994).

Trauma to teeth and periodontal disease also varied by social class amongst children. For example trauma to teeth, which affected 17% of 8–15-year-olds in 1993, is more common in lower social classes, though this trend appears to be changing (O'Brien 1994).

In adults

The inequalities in oral health are less marked than in children. In the national survey of 1988 there was a marked variation in the social class spread of edentulousness; for example 14% of social classes I, II, and IIINM had no remaining natural teeth compared with 32% of social classes IV and V. The inequalities in oral health were not as pronounced in the dentate. In social classes IIIM, IV and V 41% had 18 or more sound and unfilled teeth compared to 33% of social classes I, II, and IIINM (Todd and Lader 1991). In between 1978 and 1988 the mean numbers of decayed/unsound teeth had decreased more in social classes IV and V (2.7 to 1.8) compared to higher social classes (1.5 to 0.8) (Watt and Sheiham 1999). These trends continued in the 1998 survey, which indicated that a person was almost nine times as likely to have no teeth if they had no qualification and four times higher if their qualifications were below degree level. Being from the north of Great Britain was also a factor that had an effect, with the odds of having no teeth rising as distance from the south of England increased (Treasure *et al.* 2001).

With respect to periodontal disease, people who come from higher social backgrounds, have greater levels of education attainment, reside in urban areas, or are female, had less periodontal disease than males who are less educated and live in rural areas (Todd and Lader 1991; Watt and Sheiham 1999). While oral cancers are rare in the UK, males living in deprived areas appeared to be more susceptible (Watt and Sheiham 1999).

Amongst ethnic minorities

Watt and Sheiham (1999) concluded that there were no differences in oral health among ethnic minorities when groups of the same social class were compared. The authors suggested that ethnicity as a variable might not be relevant any longer and might distract attention from more important variables such as social class and incomes.

National, regional, and district inequalities

There are considerable inequalities in oral health status between children and adults living in the poorer north of England and the wealthier south of England. In the UK there is a threefold difference in the dental health of

5-year-olds resident in the north compared to 5-year-olds resident in the south of England. The regional and district inequalities are related to deprivation (Jones 2001). The regional inequalities are also seen in adults, particularly in relation to edentulousness: 19% of females resident in southeast England are edentulous compared to 33% in the north of England (Todd and Lader 1991).

Inequalities by gender

There are no differences by gender in the proportion of adult males and females who are dentate. Females have more fillings across all age bands; they have less periodontal disease but are more likely to be edentulous (Watt and Sheiham 1999).

CONCLUSIONS

There have been dramatic improvements in oral health across all age groups in the UK. There are, however, marked inequalities between children's' oral health, associated with social class and area of residence. These inequalities persist into adulthood but are less pronounced except in relation to edentulousness.

New concepts in relation to the epidemiology and management of periodontal disease suggest that there needs to be a rethink in relation to the provision of care. The efficacy of scale and polishing and calculus removal has been questioned. Periodontal disease does not appear to have a significant impact on oral health. There is a strong association between plaque and tobacco use in the aetiology of periodontal disease.

Oral cancers are rare in the UK, but the incidence and prevalence is increasing in males. There is a 50% survival rate at 5 years. Development of oral cancer is linked to smoking, alcohol use, and deficiencies in certain vitamins.

The incidence of dental caries is continuing to drop, but there are indications that this decline may have slowed in 5-year-olds. Studies demonstrate a reduction in provision of restorative care for children. Adults are retaining more natural teeth into later life. This has implications for the maintenance of their dentition.

The treatment of root caries may soon account for more restorative care than the treatment of caries in 5-year-olds. There is evidence that new concepts in diagnosis and management of dental caries has not penetrated clinical practice. However, the development of adhesive materials (which are technique sensitive) have the potential to stimulate a non-invasive approach to the management of early carious lesions. The declines in dental caries have been attributed to widespread use of fluoridated toothpastes. There is potential for further declines by reducing sugar consumption, appropriate exposure to fluorides, and appropriate use of fissure sealants.

Malocclusion does not contribute to poor oral health; its impacts lie in the social and psychological domains of health. The decision to seek orthodontic care is complex and there is evidence that dentists are often the instigators of a need not previously felt by the patient. A review of the provision of orthodontic care in the General Dental Service demonstrated that 21% of cases were unimproved or worse as a result of orthodontic treatment.

Erosion has been linked with the consumption of demineralizing food and drinks. It appears to have low prevalence at present but will need to be monitored over the next few years.

REFERENCES

Al-Dlaigan, Y. H., Shaw, L. Smith, A. (2001) Dental Erosion in a group of British 14-year-old children. Part II: Influence of dietary intake. *British Dental Journal*, 190, 258–61.

Boyle, P., McFarlane, G., and Scully, C. (1993). Oral cancer: necessity for prevention strategies. *Lancet*, **342**, 1129.

Brook P. H. and Shaw, W. C. (1989). The development of an orthodontic treatment priority index. *European Journal of Orthodontics*, **11**, 09–320.

Burt, B. (1988). The status of epidemiological data on periodontal disease. In *Periodontology today* (ed. B. Guggenheim), pp. 250–7. Basel, Kerger.

Cancer Research Campaign (2000). *CRC Cancerstats: Oral-UK*, London, Cancer Research Campaign.

Downer M. C. (1991). Improving dental health of United Kingdom adults and prospects for the future. *British Dental Journal*, **170**, 154–8.

Downer M. C. (1994). The 1993 national survey of children's dental health: a commentary on the preliminary report. *British Dental Journal*, **176**, 209–14.

Elderton R. J. (1987). Preventively orientated restorations and restorative procedures. In *Positive dental prevention* (ed. R. J. Elderton), pp. 85–115. London, Heinemann.

Elderton, R. J. (1990) *Evolution in Dental Care* Bristol, Clinical Press.

Elderton, R. (1996). The future of dentistry: treating restorative dentistry to health. *British Dental Journal*, **181**, 220–5.

Elderton, R. J. and Davies, J. A. (1984). Restorative dental treatment in the General Dental Service in Scotland, *British Dental Journal*, **157**, 196–200.

Frandsen, A. (1986). Mechanical oral hygiene practices: In *Dental plaque control measures and oral hygiene practices* (ed. H. Coe and D. V. Kleinmon), pp. 47–68. Oxford, IRL Press.

Goodson, J., Tamer, A., Haffajee, A., *et al.* (1982). Patterns of progression and digression of advanced destructive periodontal disease. *Journal of Clinical Periodontology*, **9**, 472–81.

Gray, P. G., Todd, J. E., Slack, G. L., and Bulman, J. S. (1970). *Government social survey: adult dental health in England and Wales in 1968*. London, HMSO.

Gregory, J., Lowe, S., Bates, C. J., *et al.* (2000). *National Diet and Nutrition Survey: young people aged 4 to 18 years. Volume 1: Report of the diet and nutrition survey*. London, The Stationery Office.

Hinds, K. and Gregory, J. (1995). *National Diet and Nutrition Survey: children aged $1\frac{1}{2}$ to $4\frac{1}{2}$ Years. Volume 12: Report of the Dental Survey*. London, HMSO.

Jenkins, W. (1996). The prevention and control of chronic periodontal disease. In *Prevention of oral disease* (ed. J. J. Murray), pp. 118–138. Oxford, Oxford University Press.

Jones, C. M. (2001) Capitation registration and social deprivation in England. An inverse 'dental' care Law? *British Dental Journal* 190, 203–6

Kayser, A. F. (1981). Shortened dental arches and oral function. *Journal of Oral Rehabilitation*, **8**, 457–62.

Kelly, M., Steele, J., Nuttal, N. *et al.* (2000). *Adult Dental Health Survey: oral health in the United Kingdom in 1998*. London, The Stationery Office.

Kidd, E. A. M. (1996). The carious lesion in enamel. In *Prevention of oral disease* (ed. J. J. Murray), pp. 95–106. Oxford, Oxford University Press.

Murray, J. J. and Pitts, N. B. (1997). Trends in oral health. In *Community oral health* (ed. C. Pine), pp. 126–46. Oxford, Wright.

Nadanovsky, P. and Sheiham, A. (1995). The relative contribution of dental services to the changes in caries levels of 12-year-old children in 18 industrialised countries in the 1970s and early 1980s. *Community Dentistry and Oral Epidemiology*, **23**, 231–9.

Nunn J., Morris, J., Pine, C., *et al.* (2001). The condition of teeth in the UK in 1998 and implications for the future. *British Dental Journal*, **189**, 639–44.

O'Brien, M. (1994). *Children's dental health in the UK 1993*. London, HMSO.

Palmer, J. D. and Pitts, N. B. (1994). Child dental health – is it still good news? *British Dental Journal*, **177**, 235–57.

Pilot, T. (1997). Public health aspects of oral diseases and disorders: periodontal disease. In *Community oral health* (ed. C. Pine), pp. 82–3. Oxford, Wright.

Pitts, N. B., Fyffe, H. E., and Nugent, Z. (1995). The Scottish Health Boards Epidemiological Programme. Report of the 1994/5 Survey of 14-year-old children. University of Dundee. Quoted in J. J. Murray and N. B. Pitts (1997), 'Trends in oral health'. In *Community oral health* (ed. C. Pine), pp. 126–46. Oxford, Wright.

Pitts, N. B., Evans, D. J. Nugent, Z. J., *et al.* (1999). The dental caries experience of 5-year-old children in the United Kingdom. Surveys co-ordinated by the British Association for the Study of Community Dentistry in 1997/98. *Community Dental Health*, **16**(1), 50–6.

Rugg-Gunn A., Carmichael, C. L., and Ferrell, R. S. (1984). Relationship between dietary habits and caries increment assessed over two years in 405 English school children. *Archives Oral Biology*, **29**, 983–92.

Shaw, W. C. (1997). Dento facial irregularities. In *Community oral health* (ed. C. Pine), pp. 104–11. Oxford, Wright.

Sheiham, A. (1991). Why sugar consumption should be below 15 kg per person in industrialised countries: the dental evidence. *British Dental Journal*, **171**, 63–5.

Socransky, S., Haffajee, A., Goodson, J., and Linde, J. (1984). New concepts of destructive periodontal disease. *Journal of Clinical Periodontology*, **11**, 21–32.

Stell, P. and McCormick, M. (1985). Cancer of the head and neck: are we doing any better? *Lancet*, **11**, 1127.

Sreebny, L. M. (1982). Sugar availability, sugar consumption and dental caries. *Community Dentistry and Oral Epidemiology*, **10**, 1–7.

Steele, J. G., Sheiham, A., Marcenes, W., and Walls, A. W. G. (1998). Diet and nutrition in Great Britain: an edited summary from Volume 2: Report of the Oral Health Survey of the National Diet and Nutrition Survey: people aged 65 years and over commissioned by the Department of Health. *Gerodontology*, **15**, 99–106.

Todd, J. (1975). *Children's dental health in England and Wales 1973*. London, HMSO.

Todd, J. E. and Dodd, T. (1985). *Children's dental health in the UK 1983*. London, HMSO.

Todd, J. E. and Lader, D. (1991). *Adult dental health, 1988, UK*. London, HMSO.

Treasure, E., Kelly, M. Nuttall, N., *et al.* (2001). Factors associated with oral health: a multivariate analysis of results from the 1998 Adult Dental Health survey. *British Dental Journal*, **190** (2), 60–8.

Watt, R. and Sheiham, A. (1999). Inequalities in oral health: a review of the evidence and recommendations for action. *British Dental Journal*, **187**, 6–12.

Whitehead, M. (1991). The concepts and principles of equity and health. *Health Promotion International*, **6**, 217–26.

FURTHER READING

Murray, J. J. (1996). The changing pattern of dental disease. In *Prevention of oral disease*, 3rd edn (ed. J. J. Murray), pp. 250–66. Oxford, Oxford University Press.

Murray, J. J. and Pitts, N. (1997). Trends in oral health. In *Community oral health* (ed. C. Pine), pp. 126–46. Oxford, Wright.

USEFUL WEBSITES

Dental Health Services Research Unit at Dundee maintains the BASCD data: www.dundee.ac.uk/dhsru/CDH

Department of Health: www.doh.gov.uk

7 Evidence-based dentistry

CONTENTS

By the end of this chapter you should be able to:

- Define the terms evidence-based medicine (EBM) and evidence-based dentistry (EBD).
- Describe the reasons for the development of EBM and EBD.
- Understand the nomenclature of EBD.
- Implement an EBD approach to a clinical problem.
- Begin using EBD as part of your own continuing education.

This chapter links with:
- Introduction to the principles of public health (Chapter 1).
- Public health approaches to prevention and treatment (Chapter 4).
- Overview of epidemiology (Chapter 5).
- Critical appraisal of literature (Chapter 8).
- Prevention in practice: caries, periodontal disease, and oral cancers (Chapters 12, 14, and 15).

INTRODUCTION

In the mid-1970s various writers began to question the domination of the medical model of health. Ivan Illich (1997) claimed that health services actually disabled people from normal coping with illness because medicine led people to expect a magic bullet for every ailment. Thomas McKeown (1976) questioned the role of medicine in the decline of communicable diseases in the UK. He found that the declines in the incidence and prevalence of communicable diseases had occurred before their microbial cause had been identified and *before* an effective clinical intervention had been developed. McKeown attributed the declines to better nutrition and improved housing conditions, which had deteriorated at the beginning of the Industrial Revolution.

But Archie Cochrane (1972) went further: he questioned whether many clinical interventions (although long established) were indeed effective or efficient. He suggested that doctors were more prone to act on the basis of 'medical opinion' rather than their knowledge of scientific fact.

At this time there were also concerns about the rising costs of health care services. It became imperative that money was seen to be spent on 'effective' interventions. Patients' views were also a factor in the desire to evaluate the outcomes of clinical practice. Consumers of health care wanted to be sure that the treatments they were asked to undergo had some chance of success. Increasingly clinicians themselves wanted the best possible evidence on which to base their clinical decisions and actions (Sackett and Rosenberg 1995). But, while considerable resources are spent on clinical research, little has been spent on the implementation of research evidence into clinical care (McClone *et al.* 2001).

The introduction of a 'problem-based learning' approach to clinical education, first developed at McMaster Medical School in Canada, stimulated new thinking in addressing solutions to clinical problems. Students became responsible for their own learning and were encouraged to solve clinical problems through self-directed learning rather than by accepting the didactic teaching of 'experts'. Short- and long-term evaluation of problem-based learning suggests that those exposed to it show substantial improvements in their ability to 'generate and defend clinical and management decisions' (Sackett and Rosenberg 1995), and that they retain those skills after qualification and during time spent in the real world of clinical practice.

WHAT IS EBM?

EBM has been defined as the 'ability to track down, critically appraise (for its validity and usefulness), and incorporate a rapidly growing body of evidence into clinical practice' (Sackett and Rosenberg 1995). The rise of clinical trials, particularly the so-called gold standard 'randomized controlled trial' (RCT) (see Chapter 5)), means that there is now an abundance of evidence with the potential to inform medical practice. Sackett and Rosenberg (1995), however, have questioned whether it is being implemented in the 'front line' of patient care. They summarized doctors' views of the barriers to implementing EBM as: no time to read, out of date text books and poorly organized journal libraries. But no matter how good the research evidence is, it must be combined with clinical experience. Neither is sufficient alone (Sackett and Rosenberg 1995)

WHAT IS EBD?

EBD has been defined as a 'process that restructures the way in which we think about clinical problems' and is characterized by 'making decisions based on known evidence' (Richards and Lawrence 1995). The Schanschieff report (1986) identified the problem of inappropriate treatment in the General Dental Service in the UK as being due to dentists not keeping up to date with new developments. There is a problem in dentistry with the amount of reliable evidence available (Jokstad 1998; Richards and Lawerence 1995). There is therefore a need to develop the skills of EBD amongst dentists and to gather more reliable evidence on which to base clinical practice.

How to do EBD

Figure 7.1 illustrates the main stages in the process of EBD, as described by Richards and Lawrence (1995).

Identifying the clinical problem

The first, and perhaps the most important step in EBD is asking a clear question about a clinical problem. The question must be relevant to the patient's problem and phrased in such a way that it will point you towards relevant and accurate answers (Sackett and Rosenberg 1995).

Table 7.1 describes a number of stages in developing your clinical question in order to elicit the best search results (after Sackett 1996). Look at it for a while and then attempt to develop your own clinical question about a problem you have encountered.

Now that you have established what your question is, the next stage is to search for evidence. Evidence can be derived from a number of sources: it may be on an individual basis, what you have observed (signs and symptoms of a patient who has the condition), or on the basis of research evidence where a variety of clinical interventions on populations of patients is reported upon (Richards and Lawerence 1995).

Locating the evidence

Richards and Lawrence (1995) suggest that there are four basic routes to finding the evidence: ask an expert, read a textbook, find the relevant article in your reprint file, or search a database such as MEDLINE.

Asking an expert is a good starting point, but they may not be completely aware of all the up-to-date evidence, and often hold quite subjective opin-

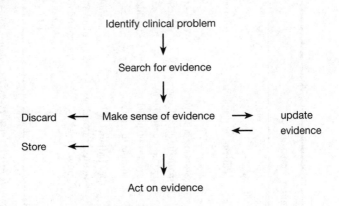

Reproduced with permission from: Richards, D and Lawrence, A 1995. Evidence based dentistry. British Dental Journal 1995; 179:270-273

Figure 7.1 The process of using EBD to make clinical decisions. (Reproduced from Richards and Lawrence 1995 with permission. See Permissions.)

Table 7.1 Framing a question

Stages	1	2	3	4
Directing the Question	Patient or problem	Intervention	Comparison/intervention	Outcomes
Tips for Building	Starting with your patient, ask: 'How would I describe a groups of patients similar to mine?'	Ask yourself: 'Which main intervention am I considering?'	Ask yourself: 'What is the main alternative to compare with the intervention?'	Ask yourself: 'What can I hope to achieve or what could this exposure really affect?'
Example	'in patients with acute necrotizing gingivitis...'	'...would adding metroniadozole to standard mechanical debridement for AUG...?'	'...when compared with standard mechanical debridement alone...?'	'...lead to a faster resolution of the condition? ... Is this worth the inconvenience of taking the medication and any side effects...?'

Modified from Sackett (2002): UK Cochrane website. Reproduced with permission. See Permissions.

ions about particular issues. Reading a textbook seems like a good idea, but there is evidence that they rapidly go out of date, even when new (Altman 1991). Finding the relevant article in your reprint file sounds a good idea, but you may not have a relevant reprint and even if you do you never get around to reading it properly. Searching a database would appear to be the best way to gather the evidence, as it will be the most up to date and quite comprehensive. Access to the literature via the Internet is a simple procedure, but there is a danger of becoming swamped with articles that are not necessarily relevant or scientifically sound. This returns us to our first point: the importance of framing our question as accurately as possible.

Hierarchy of evidence

There is a recognized hierarchy in the assessment of what constitutes good evidence. Box 7.1 describes this research evidence in more detail.

Box 7.1 Hierarchy of evidence

A systematic review and meta-analyses. Systematic reviews collate existing information and generate data to establish whether 'scientific findings are consistent and can be generalized across populations settings and treatment variations'. The studies are graded according to pre-determined criteria and a conclusion for the study is assigned. This may be weighted depending on the size of the study. A final single estimate of clinical effectiveness is then produced.

An *RCT* involves participants being allocated by the flip of a coin to either one intervention (e.g. drug) or another (e.g. placebo). The groups are followed up over a period of time and then assessed on the basis of previously agreed outcomes, which were formulated at the beginning of the experiment. RCTs are believed to be the gold standard of clinical research. A fuller description of study design is provided in the epidemiology chapters of this book.

A *longitudinal cohort study* involves following two or more groups who have been selected on the basis of their exposure to a known agent, for example sugar. They are followed for a long period (reflecting the amount of time the disease may take to develop) and the outcomes are assessed and related to the known exposure to the agent. The Vipeholm study is one of the classic, albeit controversial, examples of a longitudinal cohort study in dentistry.

A *case-control study* involves matching patients with a particular disease with 'controls' in the population who have some other disease. Data are then collected on their past medical history particularly in relation to their exposure to a possible causal agent for the disease.

A *cross-sectional study* involves collecting data at a single time (getting a snapshot of time), and it will provide data such as 'the mean DMFT of 12-year-olds in 1993'.

A *case report* would describe the medical or dental history of a single patient.

(Modified from Greenhalgh 1997. Reproduced with permission. See Permissions)

There is a need to review research evidence systematically and keep up to date as new evidence emerges. The UK Cochrane centre was established in 1992 in Oxford, and its specific role is to 'collaborate with others to build, maintain and disseminate a database of systematic, up-to-date reviews of randomized controlled trials of health care' (website: www.cochrane.org.uk).

In 1993, the Cochrane Collaboration was founded. This is an international organization that aims to help people make well-informed decisions about health care by preparing, maintaining, and disseminating systematic reviews of health care effects (Alderson 1998).

In the UK there is also the NHS Centre for Reviews and Dissemination based at the University of York. This has two roles:
- to proactively carry out reviews on health care issues with respect to the NHS (e.g. effectiveness of interventions);
- to disseminate the results of research to the NHS to enhance effective decision-making.

Systematic reviews are the cornerstone of EBD. They are a review of the literature, following a strict scientific protocol that states which studies will be included, which excluded, how they will be examined and, if possible, how they will be combined to give an estimate of the overall effect of an intervention; that is, a meta-analysis. There are two websites which are very useful for dentists to check to see if a review has been undertaken on the area in which they are interested:
- The Cochrane Collaboration (www.som.flinders.edu.au/fusa/cochrane.html), where the reviews are usually limited to RCTs.
- The NHS Centre for Reviews and Dissemination (www.york.ac.uk/inst/crd).

A systematic review can be difficult to read and interpret, and it may be worth searching for a published summary paper of the review using the authors' names from the main review.

Making sense of the evidence

Once you have gathered your material, the next stage is to appraise it and see if it makes a contribution to 'good' evidence about your problem. Chapter 8 deals in more detail with making sense of the evidence. After you have appraised the material, you decide to discard it, or keep it. Should you keep it is important to constantly update the material.

The busy practitioner may feel overwhelmed with the approach described above and may ask the question: 'Why has someone else not looked at the evidence for me?' In some cases this has been done and the evidence has been published, but it is very important to understand the types of ways in which this may have been undertaken.

Various initiatives are available in the United Kingdom to assist with this. For example the Database of Abstracts of Reviews of Effectiveness (DARE) (website: www.agatha.york.ac.ik/darehp.html) includes structured abstracts of systematic reviews which have been critically appraised by the NHS Centre for Reviews and Dissemination.

The Cochrane Collaboration Oral Health Group (www.cochrane-oral.man.ac.uk) makes contributions to the Cochrane library and maintains a database of reviews of relevance to oral health.

Evidence-based guidelines for practice are published by SIGN (Scottish Intercollegiate Guidelines Network: www.sign.ac.uk) and are available on their website. These guidelines have been produced-based on the best possible evidence, but they are presented without the evidence.

In contrast, in Wales, a series of Health Evidence Bulletins have been produced, one of which is on oral health (NHS Wales 1998). This bulletin covers a wide range of subjects and supplies references to support the statements made. It uses two classifications to aid the description of the statements made: one for the level of evidence, and the other for the potential benefit to health. Boxes 7.2 and 7.3 summarize the classifications.

When discussing tooth decay, the Welsh bulletin gives the use of both fluoride varnishes and fluoride mouth-rinses a **1** for health gain, but while varnish receives both a **I** and a **V** for evidence, mouth-rinses only receive a **V**. This suggests that the evidence supporting the use of varnishes is considerably stronger than mouthwashes.

Box 7.2 Types of evidence

Type I At least one good systematic review (including at least one RCT).
Type II At least one good RCT.
Type III Well-designed interventional studies without randomization.
Type IV Well-designed observational studies.
Type V Expert opinion, influential reports, and studies.

Box 7.3 Potential benefit to health

Beneficial (1) Effectiveness clearly demonstrated.
Likely to be beneficial (2) Effectiveness not so firmly established.
Trade-off between beneficial and adverse effects (3) Effects weighed according to individual circumstances.
Unknown (4) Insufficient/inadequate for recommendation.
Unlikely to be beneficial (5) Ineffectiveness is not as clearly demonstrated as for 6.
Likely to be ineffective or harmful (6) Ineffectiveness or harm clearly demonstrated.

DISCUSSION POINTS

Choose a clinical procedure that you have undertaken in the last month. Search for guidelines and other summary evidence. How does the care you provided match up to the evidence you found? What would you do differently (if anything) next time?

Acting on the evidence

This is the final phase of EBD, introducing it to front-line clinical practice and disseminating the evidence as widely as possible.

DOES EBM WORK?

Recent evaluations of EBM suggest that there are three ways in which a clinician can be kept up to date (Sackett 1995):

1. Learning how to practice EBM.
2. Seeking and applying EBM summaries produced by others.
3. Accepting evidence-based protocols produced by colleagues.

There is evidence that clinicians who were trained with a problem-based learning approach to medicine keep up to date for longer than their colleagues who were not trained with problem-based learning in relation to EBM. The former were also shown to be more content clinicians (Sackett 1995).

There are problems with EBD in that there is not enough reliable evidence at present on which to base clinical decisions. In addition, there are barriers to dentists incorporating new evidence into their clinical practice. McClone *et al.* (2001) has summarized these barriers as: knowledge and attitude of the practitioner (e.g. out-of-date knowledge), patient factors, practice environment, educational environment, wider health system (e.g. lack of financial incentives), and the social environment (e.g. media influencing demand for treatment). In order to effectively incorporate new evidence, imaginative ways will need to be sought to overcome these very different barriers.

EBM: A NOTE OF CAUTION

The implications of some interpretations of EBM is that if evidence is not deduced then it is inferior. Most qualitative research would never be considered as part of the hierarchy of evidence in EBM. Giacomini (2001) argues that while quantitative and qualitative research are distinctive, they both rely on systematic empirical observations and both generate empirical evidence.

Clinicians can therefore gain new insights from qualitative research which are not available in quantitative research. On a similar theme, Greenhalgh has suggested that while EBM may be used to inform clinical decision-making, the actual process (the one-to-one between the doctor and the patient) where a doctor applies his/her clinical competency 'lacks rules that can be generally and unconditionally applied to every case, even every case of single disease' (Greenhalgh 1999). So, EBM cannot explain everything. Most of the evidence is derived in populations and then applied in individual surgeries, bearing in mind the patient's individual characteristics. This interpretative process cannot always be defined within the guidelines of the evidence base.

CONCLUSION

EBD involves the systematic collection and incorporation of research evidence into clinical practice, to improve the quality and effectiveness of interventions for consumers and providers of health care. It has implications for the delivery of health care at both the individual and community level. This chapter has briefly reviewed how EBD is done and described the sources of evidence and hierarchy of evidence available.

REFERENCES

Alderson, P. (1998). The Cochrane Collaboration: an introduction. *Evidence-Based Dentistry*, **1**, 25–6.

Altman, D. (1991). *Practical statistics for medical research*. London, Chapman and Hall.

Cochrane, A. L. (1972). *Effectiveness and efficiency: random reflections on health services.* London, Nuffield Provincial Hospitals Trust.

Cochrane, A. L. (1989). Foreword. In *Effective care in pregnancy and childbirth* (ed.), pp. XX–XX. Oxford University Press.

Giacomini, M. K. (2001). The rocky road: qualitative research as evidence. *Evidence Based Medicine*, 2001, **6**, 4–6.

Greenhalgh, T. (1997). Education and Debate: How to read a paper: getting your bearings (deciding what the paper is about). *British Medical Journal*, **315**, 243–6.

Greenhalgh, T. (1999). Education and Debate: Narrative based medicine in an evidence based world. *British Medical Journal*, **317**, 323–5.

Guyatt, G., Jaeschke, R., Heddle,N., *et al.* (1995). 2: Interpreting study results: confidence intervals. *Canadian Medical Association*, **152**, 169–73.

Illich, I. (1977). *Limits to Medicine*. London, Penguin.

Jokstad, A. (1998). Editorial: Evidence-based healthcare: avoiding ivory tower research? *Evidence-Based Dentistry*, **1**, 5–6.

McClone, P., Watt, R., and Sheiham, A. (2001). Opinion: Evidence-based dentistry: an overview of the challenges in changing professional practice. *British Dental Journal*, **190**, 636–9.

McKeown, T. (1976). *The modern rise of populations*. London, Arnold.

NHS Wales (1998). *Oral health*. Cardiff, Health Evidence Bulletins.

Richards, D. and Lawrence, A. (1995). Evidence based dentistry. *British Dental Journal*, **179**, 270–3.

Sackett, D. and Rosenberg, W. (1995). Guest editorial: On the need for evidence-based medicine. *Health Economics*, 4, 249–54.

Sackett, D., Richardson, W. S., Rosenberg, WMC *et al* (1996). *Evidence-based medicine: how to practice and teach EBM.* London, Churchill Livingstone.

Schanschieff Report (1986) *Report of the Committee of Enquiry into unnecessary Dental Treatment*, London, HMSO.

FURTHER READING

Altman, D. (1991). *Practical statistics for medical research*. London, Chapman and Hall.
Greenhalgh, T. (1997). Education and Debate: How to read a paper: the Medline database. *British Medical Journal*, **315**, 180–3.
Greenhalgh, T. (1997). Education and Debate: How to read a paper: getting your bearings (deciding what the paper is about). *British Medical Journal*, **315**, 243–6.
Greenhalgh, T. (1997). Education and Debate: How to read a paper: papers that summarise other papers (systematic reviews and meta analyses). *British Medical Journal*, **315**, 672–5.
Greenhalgh, T. (1997). Education and Debate: How to read a paper: papers that go beyond numbers (qualitative research). *British Medical Journal*, **315**, 740–3.

USEFUL WEBSITES

The Cochrane Collaboration: www.som.flinders.edu.au/fusa/cochrane.html
The Cochrane Collaboration Oral Health Group: www.cochrane-oral.man.ac.uk
Database of Abstracts of Reviews of Effectiveness (DARE): www.agatha.york.ac.ik/darehp.html
NHS Centre for Reviews and Dissemination based at the University of York: www.york.ac.uk/inst/crd
Scottish Intercollegiate Guidelines Network: www.sign.ac.uk
The UK Cochrane centre at the University of Oxford: www.ox.ac.uk/cochrane

8 Critical appraisal of literature

CONTENTS

By the end of this chapter you should be able to:

- Define the term 'critical appraisal'.
- Give reasons why the literature needs to be appraised.
- Describe how to undertake the critical appraisal of an article in a scientific journal.
- Describe some key statistical considerations in good study design.

This chapter links with:
- Public health approaches to prevention (Chapter 4).
- Oral epidemiology (Chapters 5–8).
- Evidence-based dentistry (Chapter 7).
- Prevention in practice: caries, periodontal disease and oral cancer (Chapters 12, 14, 15).

INTRODUCTION

You will come across a plethora of scientific material as part of your dental training. It may be in the form of journal articles, textbooks, lecture notes, advertising leaflets from dental companies, or clinical advice from a tutor in a teaching clinic. Some of this information may be conflicting and/or misleading. How will you know whether you are receiving sound scientific evidence or someone's uninformed opinion? You cannot assume that an article appearing in a respected, peer-reviewed medical journal contains reliable information (Altman 2000).

Most of what appears in the dental journals are 'follow-up' or 'retrospective' studies, and there is in fact little solid evidence for the majority of therapeutic interventions (Jokstad 1998). While these studies do contribute to clinical practice, the clinical importance would be vastly improved if a study were designed prospectively to answer a specific clinical question.

It is essential that clinicians working with either individual patients or in the community base their decisions and actions on the best possible evidence in order to improve and advance clinical practice (Sackett and Rosenberg 1995). At a time of scarce resources it is important that money is spent on clinically effective interventions. Critical appraisal is a core element of evidence-based medicine and evidence-based dentistry.

While it is not within the scope of this text to deal with critical appraisal in detail, some important aspects in reading the literature will be highlighted so you can begin the process. In order to improve your skills and competency we advise you to read the excellent texts and papers we recommend under further reading at the end of this chapter.

CRITICAL APPRAISAL

Critical appraisal has been described as assessing the quality of the methodology used to investigate a problem (Greenhalgh 1997). Within the context of dentistry it has been described as making sense of the evidence and systematically considering its validity, results, and relevance to dentistry (Richards and Lawrence 1995).

How to critically appraise a scientific paper

Greenhalgh (1997) has identified three key questions you should ask yourself when reading a scientific paper (reproduced in Box 8.1).

While most articles in scientific journals now take the IMRAD format (see Box 8.2), the most important criterion for choosing to read a paper should be the quality of the methods section (Greenhalgh 1997).

It is a useful practice to employ a logical approach when learning to critically appraise a paper. Start with the **title** of the article and ask yourself if it gives you a good idea of the material covered in the paper. Sometimes it is helpful to turn the title into a question so you can more easily grasp why the authors undertook the study.

Box 8.1 Key questions for critical appraisal

1. Why was the study done, and what clinical question were the authors addressing?
2. What type of study was done?
3. Was this design appropriate to the research?

(Modified from Greenhalgh 1997.)

Box 8.2 IMRAD formal

I   Introduction (Why was the research done?)
M   Methods (How the study was done and how were the results analysed?)
R   Results (What results were obtained?)
D   Discussion (What do the results mean?)

(Modified from Greenhalgh 1997.)

Next look at the **abstract**, if there is one. It should give a clear and concise account of the aims and objectives of the study and a brief synopsis of the methods used, including selection of sample and sample size, important variables, and a summary of the important results, which inform the discussion and conclusions.

The **introduction** should tell you why the study was undertaken and provide you with an introduction to the topic. You should be able to say what type of paper it is. For example, is it a review article, a case report, a clinical trial? Ask yourself if it has built on the existing literature in the field in a logical and sequential fashion? Are there any omissions of key papers in the field? Are the aims and objectives clearly stated? If not, how might they be better stated?

The **materials and methods** section is key to critical appraisal. Was the design of the study appropriate to the research? The methodology should be explicit: it should be like a recipe, and the reader should be in a position to say why the study was done, how it was done, where it was done, what was done, and to whom (Plamping 1986).

Box 8.3 Methodology checklist

- Why was the study undertaken?
- How was it done?
- Where was it done?
- What was done?
- To whom was it done?

(Plamping 1986.)

There are two types of study (Greenhalgh 1997):
- *Primary*, which reports on research first hand.
- *Secondary*, which summarizes and attempts to draw conclusions from other primary studies.

Certain types of investigations require specific study designs. Box 8.4 describes a broad categorization of research and suggests the most appropriate study design for its investigation. There is also the hierarchy of evidence as discussed in the chapters on Epidemiology (p. 5) and Evidence-based dentistry (p. 7).

When designing the methodology authors should consider how the results will be eventually analysed. Provision should also be made for *confounding* variables. Any observational study that compares populations by a particular variable (e.g. uses betel nut, does not use betel nut) and then attributes the observed differences found in another variable (e.g. oral cancer rates) to that particular variable may not have considered some other confounding variables. Age and gender are the most common confounding variables in health-related research (Moles and dos Santos Silva 2001).

DISCUSSION POINTS

An observational study is planned to compare oral cancer incidence and betel nut use in a population. What confounding variables should be considered?

Box 8.4 Broad fields of research

Therapy (testing the efficacy of a clinical intervention): the preferred study design is the *randomized controlled trial.*

Diagnosis (testing whether a new test is reliable and valid): the preferred study design is a *cross-sectional survey.*

Screening: the preferred study design is a *cross-sectional survey.*

Prognosis (following patients whose disease is picked up at an early stage): the study design of choice is a *longitudinal cohort study.*

Causation: the preferred study is a *cohort or case control study.*

(*Modified from Greenhalgh 1997. Reproduced with permission. See Permissions.*)

The **results** section should contain data which are clear and concise. It is a good idea to derive the results yourself should sufficient data be available. You should be satisfied that the results presented were derived from the data obtained.

Were appropriate statistical tests used? A statistical test should conform to the underlying assumptions by which the test is applied. The statistical tests used should be fairly familiar and, if not in common usage, they should be referenced and the reason for their choice and the underlying assumptions clearly stated. Statistical methods should 'be described with sufficient detail to enable a knowledgeable reader with access to the original data to verify the reported results' (Greenhalgh (1997)). This aspect will be considered in more detail in the next section.

The **discussion** is often the place in an article where the authors give full rein to their imagination. Speculation can occupy a greater amount of space than observations on the findings in the study! You should consider if the authors have managed to draw together the 'known literature' and the current findings/results derived from the paper. Any weaknesses in the study should be discussed here, particularly in relation to extrapolation of ideas or generalizability. Generalizability is an important concept: it refers to whether the results obtained can be applied to other groups and populations.

The **conclusions** should be founded on the discussion and results, and be based on empirical data derived from the study and/or in association with the existing literature.

Many papers have minor, and some may have major faults. The objective of critical appraisal is not to make spurious criticism; it is to decide whether a flaw is serious enough to compromise the methodology and therefore the results obtained, the conclusions drawn, and the generalizability of the paper and the applicability to dental practice.

Finally, remember that an unsuccessful outcome is as important to clinical practice as a successful outcome. However, many journals do have a bias towards successful reviews (Richards and Lawrence 1995).

DISCUSSION POINTS

Questions have been raised in the media about the safety of hydrogen peroxide tooth whiteners. Animal researchers in the University of Buffalo found that it may promote cancer development. Their study involved placing hydrogen peroxide on existing pre-cancerous lesions in the cheek pouches of twelve hamsters. (Source: *BDA News*, April 1999.)

Many patients in the UK have received 'whitening' treatment in the dental surgery. What would you say to a patient of yours who had read this report and was concerned?

SOME KEY CONSIDERATIONS IN THE USE OF STATISTICS

Altman (1991,1999, 2000) has suggested that a substantial number of papers published in medical journals had poor or flawed statistics. Poor statistics could lead to unreliable evidence and erroneous clinical implications. Sometimes statistics are seen by authors as a troublesome but necessary 'add-on' to get a paper published. The growth of some very good statistical software packages means that a whole battery of tests can be applied to data without any understanding of the assumptions underpinning the tests themselves. In this book it is not possible to provide a comprehensive overview of statistics; however, we have included a selection of books and articles at the end of this chapter which we have found useful. Most dentists may never find themselves writing papers but they will certainly read a lot of textbooks, papers, and scientific material in the course of their careers.

Statistics should be about common sense and good design (Altman 1991). There are a number of key statistical considerations in a good study design.

The null hypothesis

A good starting-point for any research is to assume that there is no difference between two interventions: the null hypothesis. This involves estimating the likelihood that the observed results in an experiment would have occurred by chance if the null hypothesis were true (Altman 1995). The object of the research then becomes disproving the theory of no difference (Greenhalgh 1997).

Box 8.5 Key statistical considerations in good study design

- The null hypothesis.
- Sample size and power considerations.
- Choice of sample and control of subjects.
- Design of study.
- Gathering the data.
- Presentation of data.
- Choice of statistics and summary analysis.
- Confidence intervals.

Sample size and power considerations

It is important that the sample derived to investigate the question is large enough to detect a difference of clinical importance should such a difference exist. Be wary of small sample sizes. It is possible for a statistician to work out the sample size necessary (called the power of the sample) when something is known about the variable, the standard deviation, and the size of effect which would be of clinical importance. A good paper should therefore include details of how the sample size was determined.

The choice of samples and controls

In most studies you will be looking to see if there is a representative sample of the general population, in order that the findings will generalizable. There will be important exceptions, such as cohort studies, where you are looking at people with similar exposures to a known agent. However, what becomes important in these studies are the controls. They must be matched carefully with the cohort and all known confounding variables accounted for.

Design of the study and gathering the data

In the earlier section on critical appraisal of the literature, the importance of choosing a study design appropriate to the question was stressed. Look closely at how the subjects were gathered. In a randomized controlled trial, what method of 'randomization' was used? In a cross-sectional survey, how were subjects selected? Was it opportunistic? Did subjects volunteer? What steps were taken to ensure that the data are reliable and repeatable? What steps were taken to eliminate the effects of the researcher or the research procedure on the responses of the subjects (Altman 1991; Greenhalgh 1997).

Presentation of data

This is the area of statistics most frequently abused. A good diagram or table can present material in a very concise and informative way, but equally,

---

Box 8.6 Presentation of data: common areas to look for in the literature

- Is the number of subjects clearly stated?
- Are appropriate axes labelled and scales indicated?
- Is a true zero used?
- Do the titles adequately describe the contents and graphs?
- Do graphs indicate the relevant variability?

(Modified from Altman 1991.)

---

poor presentation can mislead. Common areas to look for are summarized in the Box 8.6.

Choice of statistics and summary analysis

The choice of the statistics used and the analysis should reflect the type of study undertaken. Some common areas to look for are presented in Box 8.7.

Confidence intervals

Based on the observed result and size of the sample, a confidence interval, can be calculated. It will provide a range of probabilities within which the true probability will lie, 90 to 95% of the time. A most important advantage of the confidence interval is that it can also help determine whether a trial is definitive or not. Guyatt *et al.* (1995) suggest that if the lower boundary of the confidence interval is above the threshold considered for clinical significance, then the trial is positive and definitive. If the lower boundary is below the threshold for clinical significance then the trial is deemed positive but more studies with larger sample sizes are required. Equally, if the upper boundary of the confidence interval is below the threshold of clinical significance then the trial is negative and definitive. But if some of the upper boundary crosses the threshold of clinical

---

Box 8.7 Choice of statistics and summary analysis

- Are the underlying assumptions for the tests satisfied?
- How do you know?
- Are the results clinically significant as well as statistically significant? What is the size of the effect if clinically significant?
- Have a large number of tests been carried out which have not been reported?
- Were hypotheses generated by exploration of the data set and then confirmed using the same data set?

(Modified from Altman 1991.)

significance more trials are needed with larger sample sizes in order for the trial to be definitive.

DISCUSSION POINTS

Assume you are reading an article on the relationship between cancer mortality and fluoridation of water supplies. The study is located in 10 fluoridated and 10 non-fluoridated towns in the USA. Preliminary results suggest there was an increase of 20% in cancer mortality rate between 1950 and 1970 in fluoridated towns compared to an increase of 10% in non-fluoridated towns.

What type of study design would best investigate the relationship between cancer mortality and fluoridation of the water supplies?

What confounding variables would you expect to be considered?

Critical appraisal checklists are becoming popular, and many journals are laying down criteria for the reporting of particular types of research. The CONSORT statement presented 21 items which were required to be reported in randomized controlled trials and these items were required to be derived from empirical data whenever possible (Moher 1998). Quorum is another checklist that is being used to report systematic reviews. While checklists are important, a note of caution is required. Most medical journals are adopting the approach that papers with less than 80% follow-up will be rejected. But the assessment of good research should take account of what is possible in certain circumstances and what is achievable (Altman 2000). Studies of people trying to change their diet or stop smoking will have, by the very nature of the work, large drop-out rates. Should these studies not, therefore, be reported?

QUALITATIVE RESEARCH

Scientists generally put a high value on data they can count and apply statistical tests to. Qualitative research methodology is about 'making sense of, or interpreting phenomena in terms of the meanings people bring to them' (Greenhalgh and Taylor 1997). Qualitative research can be used to define the original research question (Jick 1997), or may be used in combination with quantitative methods (Mays and Pope 1999). The field of critical appraisal in qualitative research is not as extensive as that for quantitative research. However, qualitative research is becoming more common in mainstream medical and dental journals. Greenhalgh and Taylor (1997) have developed a number of questions (Box 8.8) which should help you determine the quality of the research you are reading. These criteria are still undergoing review, but give an indication of some of the key considerations in evaluating qualitative research.

Box 8.8 Checklist for qualitative research

- Did the paper describe an important problem with a clearly formulated question?
- Was the qualitative approach justified and appropriate to the question?
- How were the settings and people selected?
- How were the data collected? Are the methods clearly described?
- How were the data analysed? What attempts were made to ensure quality?
- Are the results credible? Are they clinically important?
- What were the conclusions? Are these conclusions justified by the results?

(Modified from Greenhalgh and Taylor 1997.)

CONCLUSIONS

Critical appraisal has been described as assessing the quality of the methodology used to investigate a problem. It is about making sense of the evidence and systematically considering its validity, results, and relevance to dentistry. Critical appraisal is a core element in evidence-based dentistry, and the more you do it, the more adept you will become at it. Challenge material you come in contact with, whatever the source. Finally, you may find the *aide-mémoire* reproduced in Box 8.9 helpful in developing your skills.

Box 8.9 What have I learned from this paper?

- To whom does this information apply?
- What causal conclusions may be drawn from it?
- How general are these conclusions?
- What previous studies does this one replicate?
- Are its results replicable?
- To what extent does it describe or bear on the 'real world'?
- What major gaps remain in my knowledge?
- How can I fill them?
- What leads (or warnings) for future researchers does the paper give?

(Modified from Altman 1991 and Greenhalgh 1997.)

REFERENCES

Altman, D. (1991). *Practical statistics for medical research*. London, Chapman and Hall.

Altman, D. (1999). Statistics in the medical literature: 3. *Statistics in Medicine*, **18**, 487–90.

Altman, D. (2000). Statistics in medical journals: some recent trends. *Statistics in Medicine*, **19**, 3275–89.

Anon (1999). Tooth whiteners, *British Dental Association News*, **13** (3).

Greenhalgh, T. (1997). How to read a paper: getting your bearings (deciding what the paper is about). [Education and Debate.] *British Medical Journal*, **315**, 243–6.

Greenhalgh, T. and Herxheimer, A. (1999). Towards a broader agenda for training in critical appraisal. *Journal of the Royal College of Physicians London*, **33**, 36–8.

Greenhalgh, T. and Taylor, R. (1997). How to read a paper: papers that go beyond numbers (qualitative research). [Education and Debate.] *British Medical Journal*, **315**, 740–3.

Guyatt, G., Jaeschke, R., Heddle, N., *et al.* (1995). 2: Interpreting study results: confidence intervals. *Canadian Medical Association*, **152**, 169–73.

International Committee of Medical Journal Editors (1997). Uniform requirements for manuscripts submitted to biomedical journals. *Annals of Internal Medicine*, **126**, 36–47.

Jick, T. (1997). Mixing quantitative and qualitative methods: triangulation in action. *Administrative Sciences Quarterly*, **24**, 602–11.

Jokstad, A. (1998). Evidence-based healthcare: avoiding ivory tower research? [Editorial.] *Evidence-Based Dentistry*, **1**, 5–6.

Mays, N. and Pope, C. (1999). *Qualitative research in health care*. London, British Medical Journal.

Moher, D. (1998). CONSORT: an evolving tool to help improve the quality of reports of randomised controlled trials. *Journal of the American Medical Association*, **279**, 1489–91.

Moher, D., Cook, D., Eastwood, S. *et al.* (1999). Improving the quality of reports of meta-analyses of randomised controlled trials: the Quorum statement. *Lancet*, **354**, 1896–900.

Moles, D. R. and dos Santos Silva, I. (2001). Causes, associations and evaluating evidence: can we trust what we read? [Toolbox.] *Evidence Based Dentistry*, **2**, 75–8.

Plamping, D. (1986). *Reviewing a paper*. Master in Dental Public Health: Study Skills Module. University College London.

Richards, D. and Lawrence, A. (1995). Evidence based dentistry. *British Dental Journal*, **179**, 270–3.

Sackett, D. and Rosenberg, W. (1995). On the need for evidence-based medicine. [Guest Editorial.] *Health Economics*, **4**, 249–54.

FURTHER READING

Altman, D. (1991). *Practical statistics for medical research*. London, Chapman and Hall.

Bulman, J. S. and Osborn, J. F. (1989). Statistics in dentistry. London, British Dental Association.

Greenhalgh, T. (1997). How to read a paper: the Medline database. [Education and Debate.] *British Medical Journal*, **315**, 180–3.

Greenhalgh, T. (1997). How to read a paper: getting your bearings (deciding what the paper is about). [Education and Debate.] *British Medical Journal*, **315**, 243–6.

Greenhalgh, T. (1997). How to read a paper: papers that summarise other papers (systematic reviews and meta analyses). [Education and Debate.] *British Medical Journal*, **315**, 672–5.

Greenhalgh, T. and Taylor, R. (1997). How to read a paper: papers that go beyond numbers (qualitative research). [Education and Debate.] *British Medical Journal*, **315**, 740–3.

Rose, G. and Barker, D. J. P. (1986). *Epidemiology for the uninitiated*. London, British Medical Association.

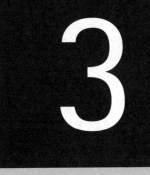

Prevention and oral health promotion

9 Principles of oral health promotion

CONTENTS

INTRODUCTION

Dental diseases affect a large number of people and cause much discomfort and pain. Their impact is therefore considerable, both to the individual and wider society (see Chapter 21 for a more detailed overview of oral health impacts). Unlike most other chronic conditions, the causes of dental diseases are well known and numerous effective preventive measures have been identified. However, treatment services dominate all oral health systems. In the UK, only a very small proportion of the NHS dental budget is spent on prevention, despite the fact that acknowledgement that treatment services will never successfully treat away the causes of dental diseases (Blinkhorn 1998).

DISCUSSION POINTS

Based upon what you have read in Chapters 1 and 2, outline the reasons why prevention is given such a low priority within the NHS?

If treatment services alone are not capable of dealing effectively with dental diseases, then other options need to be considered. Recently the health promotion movement has arisen, partly in response to the recognized limitations of treatment services to improve the health of the public. With escalating costs and wider acceptance that doctors and dentists are not able to cure most chronic conditions, increasing interest has focused on alternative means of dealing with health problems.

HISTORICAL DEVELOPMENT OF HEALTH PROMOTION

The origins of health promotion date back to the work of public health pioneers in the nineteenth century. At that time rapid industrialization led to the creation of poor and overcrowded working and living conditions for the majority of the working classes in the large industrial towns of Britain. These appalling social conditions inevitably led to epidemics of infectious disease, which spread through the population and were considered a threat to social stability. Eminent social reformers such as Edwin Chadwick and Southwood Smith highlighted the need to improve social conditions through municipal reform. In 1875 a Public Health Act was passed to control water supply, sewage disposal, and animal slaughter within industrialized towns and cities. Such measures had a significant effect on reducing the prevalence of infectious diseases long before clinical medicine had even discovered the pathogenic nature of these infections, or antibiotics.

By the late nineteenth century, as the threat of disease epidemics receded, the focus had begun to shift away from environmental measures for improving health to measures that highlighted the importance of educating individuals against the hazards of disease. This educational approach became increasingly dominated by the medical profession and as a result more disease-specific. Information campaigns, often using shock methods, were targeted at high-risk groups in an attempt to change personal habits and behaviours. The Health Education Council (later to be known as the Health Education Authority) was formed in 1968 to develop national programmes of education for the public. (In 2000 the Health Education Authority was closed down and the Health Development Agency was created.)

In 1974 the then Canadian minister of health, Marc Lalonde, published *A new perspective on the health of Canadians*, in which he argued that the major causes of death and disease were due to environmental causes, individual behaviours, and lifestyle factors rather than to biomedical characteristics (Lalonde 1974). This document was enormously influential in shifting the focus away from an individual biochemical focus to the wider public health agenda once again. It consequently led WHO to organize a series of international health promotion conferences which facilitated the development and practice of the modern health promotion movement. The first of these WHO conferences, in Ottawa in 1986, was particularly important in defining the meaning and potential of health promotion (WHO 1986).

The Ottawa Charter outlined five key areas of action as:

1. **Creating supportive environments**: recognizing the impact of the environment on health and identifying opportunities to make changes conducive to health.
2. **Building healthy public policy**: focusing attention on the impact on health of public policies from all sectors, and not just the health sector.
3. **Strengthening community action**: empowering individuals and communities in the processes of setting priorities, making decisions, and planning and implementing strategies, to achieve better health.
4. **Developing personal skills**: moving beyond the transmission of information, to promote understanding, and supporting the development of personal, social, and political skills that enable individuals to take action to promote health.
5. **Reorienting health services**: refocusing attention away from the responsibility to provide curative and clinical services towards the goal of health gain.

These key areas provide a useful range of actions to encompass the width and diversity of approaches needed in health promotion (Fig. 9.1). Later in this chapter the scope of each of these areas will be explored with reference to oral health.

DEFINITION AND PRINCIPLES OF HEALTH PROMOTION

A variety of definitions of health promotion have been proposed which highlight subtle differences in approach and emphasis. The WHO (1984) definition, however, captures the spirit and meaning well:

> Health promotion has to come to represent a unifying concept for those who recognize the need for change in the ways and conditions of living in order to promote health. Health promotion represents a mediating strategy between people and their environments, synthesizing personal choice and social responsibility in health to create a healthier future.

Health promotion has three important elements:
- Focus on tackling the determinants of health.
- Working in partnership with a range of agencies and sectors.
- Adopting a strategic approach utilizing a complementary range of actions to promote the health of the population.

Determinants of health

Health promotion focuses on the determinants of health, both the socio-economic and environmental factors, plus the individual health-related

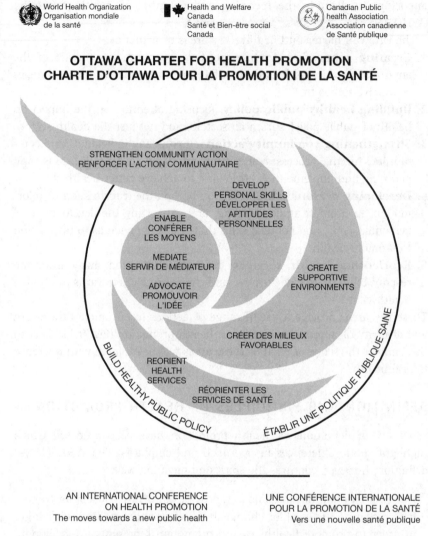

World Health Organization
Organisation mondiale
de la santé

Health and Welfare
Canada
Santé et Bien-être social
Canada

Canadian Public
health Association
Association canadienne
de Santé publique

OTTAWA CHARTER FOR HEALTH PROMOTION
CHARTE D'OTTAWA POUR LA PROMOTION DE LA SANTÉ

STRENGTHEN COMMUNITY ACTION
RENFORCER L'ACTION COMMUNAUTAIRE

DEVELOP
PERSONAL SKILLS
DÉVELOPPER LES
APTITUDES
PERSONNELLES

ENABLE
CONFÉRER
LES MOYENS

MEDIATE
SERVIR DE MÉDIATEUR

CREATE
SUPPORTIVE
ENVIRONMENTS

ADVOCATE
PROMOUVOIR
L'IDÉE

CRÉER DES MILIEUX
FAVORABLES

REORIENT
HEALTH
SERVICES

RÉORIENTER LES
SERVICES DE SANTÉ

BUILD HEALTHY PUBLIC POLICY

ÉTABLIR UNE POLITIQUE PUBLIQUE SAINE

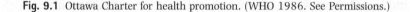

AN INTERNATIONAL CONFERENCE
ON HEALTH PROMOTION
The moves towards a new public health

November 17–21, 1986 Ottawa, Ontario, Canada

UNE CONFÉRENCE INTERNATIONALE
POUR LA PROMOTION DE LA SANTÉ
Vers une nouvelle santé publique

17–21 novembre 1986 Ottawa (Ontario) Canada

Fig. 9.1 Ottawa Charter for health promotion. (WHO 1986. See Permissions.)

behavioural elements. (See Chapter 2 for a full account of the determinants of health.) It therefore attempts to avoid a victim-blaming approach by recognizing the limited control many individuals often have over their health. In the past health professionals have ignored the complex array of factors that influence and determine human behaviour and have as a result wrongly assumed that individuals are always capable of modifying elements of their lifestyle. Such a restricted and narrow approach has most often not achieved the desired changes in behaviour. A major emphasis in health promotion is therefore *to make the healthy choices, the easy choices* by focusing attention upstream Milio (1986).

DISCUSSION POINTS

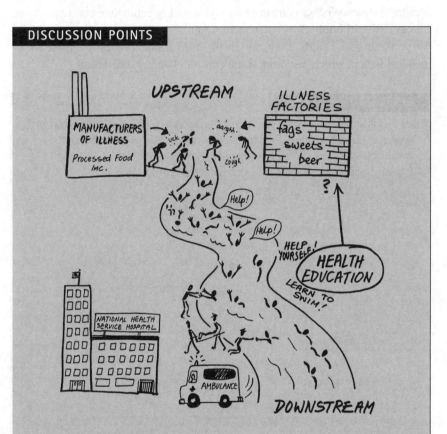

Upstream–downstream!

There I am standing by the shore of a swiftly flowing river and I hear the cry of a drowning man. So I jump into the river, put my arms around him, pull him to the shore and apply artificial respiration. Just when he begins to breathe, there is another cry for help. So I jump into the river, reach him, pull him to shore, apply artificial respiration, and then just as he begins to breathe, another cry for help. So back in the river again, without end, goes the sequence. You know I am so busy jumping in pulling them to shore, applying artificial respiration, that I have no time to see who the hell is upstream pushing them all in.

(McKinlay 1979)

In terms of health promotion what factors are working upstream creating disease in society?

As a health promoter, what are the limitations of only working downstream?

To promote oral health what would a reorientation upstream involve?

The fundamental determinants of oral health are related to the consumption of non-milk extrinsic sugars (NMES) and the effective control of plaque in the mouth. Other factors that influence oral health include optimal exposure to fluoride, and the appropriate use of good-quality dental care. The effects on oral health of excess alcohol consumption and smoking behaviour also needs to be recognized. Although all of these factors can be modified at an individual level to promote oral health, they are clearly also influenced by complex socio-political factors which are outside the control of many individuals.

DISCUSSION POINTS

The foods and drinks people select are influenced by a complex array of factors operating at varying levels. The figure below separates out these factors into individual, socio-cultural and environmental levels.
Provide at least three examples for each of these categories.

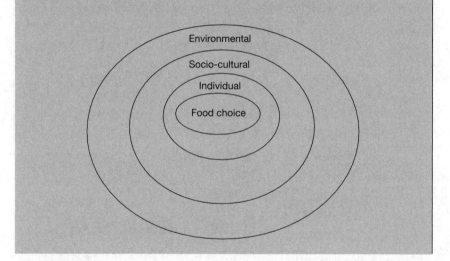

Working in partnerships

Community participation is an essential element of health promotion. The active involvement of the local community in all aspects, from the identification of the health issue to ways of initiating change, is a central principle. One of the key roles of health professionals is therefore in enabling and nurturing health promotion within communities.

By recognizing and focusing on the wide and diverse underlying determinants of health, multi-sectorial working is a key element of health promotion. Many sectors in society, for example government departments, education, agriculture, health and social services, and the voluntary sector all have a significant influence on health. It is essential that these different agencies work together to ensure that health promotion policies are established, implemented, monitored and evaluated (Box 9.1).

Box 9.1 Partners in oral health

- Health professionals, for example doctors, health visitors, pharmacists, district nurses.
- Education services, for example teachers, school governors, parents.
- Local authority staff, for example carers, planning departments, social workers, catering staff within care homes, local politicians.
- Voluntary sector, for example Age Concern, Pre-school Learning Alliance, Terrence Higgins Trust, Mind.
- Commerce and industry, for example food retailers, food producers, advertising industry, water industry.
- Government, local, national and international.

DISCUSSION POINTS

To successfully develop and implement a water fluoridation scheme within a district, describe the range of individuals and agencies that would need to be involved in the process.

Strategic action

A strategic approach is required for the development of effective health promotion policies. A strategy should be based on an appropriate assessment of local needs and resources, which enables the development of a strategic vision with clearly stated and identified aims and targets. Many health problems share common risk factors; for example, eating an unhealthy diet which is high in fat and sugars and low in fibre can lead to the development of obesity, coronary heart disease, and diabetes, as well as dental caries. Health promotion strategies based on a common risk-factor approach (Fig. 9.2) therefore offer the potential for effectively dealing with a combination of health problems together (Sheiham and Watt 2000). Not only can this prove to be more effective in the long term but it is also more efficient in the use of resources. Oral health promoters need to work closely with people in general health promotion. They have a key role of placing oral health matters on the wider health promotion agenda. (The common risk-factor approach is covered in greater detail in Chapter 2.)

Health promotion involves the population as a whole in the context of their everyday life, rather than focusing only on people at risk for specific diseases. It can attempt to influence the social norms within society by promoting the positive benefits of healthy behaviours. Health promotion can therefore utilize a combined whole-population strategy and a high-risk strategy which aims to enable people to take control over, and responsibility for, their health. (Chapter 4 outlines the features of both these approaches.)

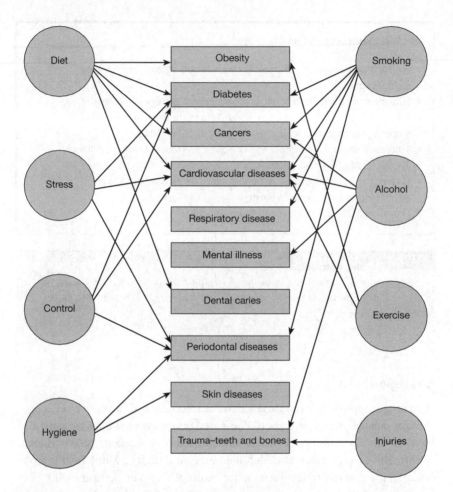

Fig. 9.2 The common risk-factor approach. (Reproduced from Sheiham and Watt 2000 with permission. See Permissions.)

DISCUSSION POINTS

Plaque levels in the population have been reduced in the last 20 years.

What factors have contributed to this decline (consider factors operating at an individual, social, and community level)?

Which of these contributory factors would you consider to be the most important explanation for the decline in plaque in the population?

ORAL HEALTH PROMOTION IN ACTION

Health promotion seeks to improve and protect health through a diverse variety of complementary strategies. The five areas for action outlined in the Ottawa Charter provide a useful structure to explore options for promoting oral health (WHO 1986).

Developing personal skills

The development of personal and social skills can be achieved through health education. Health education can be defined as opportunities created for learning specifically aimed at producing a health related goal (WHO 1984). Three basic educational objectives exist:
1. *Cognitive*: concerned with giving information and increasing knowledge.
2. *Affective*: concerned with clarifying, forming, or changing attitudes, beliefs, values, or opinions.
3. *Behavioural*: concerned with the development of skills and actions.

Essentially, then, health education aims to equip individuals and/or communities with the necessary knowledge, attitudes, and skills to maintain and improve health. Health education can therefore be considered as one of the strategies in health promotion which is specifically concerned with promoting some form of educational change.

Traditionally, dental health education has sought to increase patients' knowledge about the role of sugar and plaque in the aetiology of dental diseases. Initially such programmes were largely confined to schools. More recently oral health education has extended its aims to include activities not only directed at improvements in knowledge but also the development of appropriate oral health skills. The promotion of self-care is now seen as being of fundamental importance. Programmes are now also directed at a wider range of groups in society, for example other health and education workers and carers (Watt and Fuller 1999). (A more detailed overview of oral health education is presented in Chapter 11).

Strengthening community action

This can be achieved through developing a community development approach. This involves the mobilization of community resources, both human and material. It is a process in which the community defines its own health needs, decides how these can be best tackled, and then takes appropriate action. The advantages of this approach are that it is starting with people's concerns and is therefore likely to gain support; it focuses action on the causes of ill health identified by those affected, and the skills and confidence developed by the community can lead to sustainable improvements in health. The problems of adopting this approach include the time-consuming nature of the work, the difficulty of evaluation, and the potential conflicts that may arise within communities on setting priorities and identifying possible solutions.

Health professionals involved in community development projects need to adopt a different style of working for this approach to be successful. Rather than be the expert, they instead act as a facilitator and catalyst within the community. This requires skills in consultation, empowerment, and communication. The establishment of self-help groups, where people affected by particular oral health problems share their experiences and identify solutions, is one oral health example of community action (Fiske *et al.* 1995). A network of community cafes and food co-operatives have been established within deprived neighbourhoods in Glasgow lacking access to cheap and appealing healthy foods. Such an approach facilitates healthy food choices amongst these groups (McGlone *et al.* 1999).

Reorienting health services

The responsibility for health promotion in health services is shared among the many health professions and at the various levels of health care. All must work together towards a health care system which positively contributes to the pursuit of health. There is a need to shift resources away from the dominant treatment and curative services towards those that promote health and prevent disease. Oral health promotion is not, therefore, concerned with promoting dentistry as such. Instead, it should be involved in the development of appropriate high-quality oral care which places greater emphasis on preventive care and ways of supporting and maintaining oral health within the oral health care system.

A reorientation towards health promotion requires changes in many aspects of health services. The training and education of health professionals needs to be modified with a greater emphasis placed on the disciplines underpinning prevention and health promotion. Funding mechanisms need to encourage and reward dentists for effective prevention, and research activities should place a higher priority on health promotion agendas.

Building healthy public policy

Legislative and regulatory policy passed at either national or local level can have a very powerful influence on health by creating a social environment which protects or improves health. Thus, a key element of health promotion is placing health onto the policy agendas of influential decision-makers. One oral health example is the legislation required to fluoridate public water supplies. Another is the stricter regulation on food labelling of processed food and drink. For such future legislation to be passed dental professionals need to lobby government departments and become involved in the political processes facilitating change. Professional organizations such as the British Dental Association could follow the lead provided by medical groups and become advocates for improvements in public policy which promote oral health.

The price of products and services is a major factor determining uptake and use. Fiscal policy is a part of health promotion which seeks to influence the costs of items influential to health. At present unhealthy options are often cheaper than healthy alternatives. An important example of this is foods and drinks where European Union subsidies are currently being directed at the production of unhealthy items. Fiscal measures that reduce the costs of healthy products enable a larger number of people to select healthy options. Clearly fiscal measures in the form of taxation can also be used to increase the costs of unhealthy products, therefore making them less afford-able, the most obvious example being cigarettes. However, this may in fact increase pressure on the most disadvantaged groups in society who are often most heavily dependent on unhealthy products, and so such a move may ultimately result in a worsening of the health status of the poorest mem-bers of society (Marsh and McKay 1994).

Creating supportive environments

This aspect of health promotion recognizes the impact of the environment on health and seeks to identify opportunities to make changes conducive to better health. Healthy public policies can of course provide a legislative framework for environmental change, water fluoridation being a prime example. In addition to change at a national level, action can also take place a local level. For example, developing policies within local organizations such as schools, workplaces, and hospitals which seek to promote the health of clients and staff is an important aspect of health promotion. This approach to health promotion is termed, *organizational change*. Examples could include the establishment of non-smoking areas, exercise and chang-ing facilities, and healthy catering services where consumers can select healthy options such as sugar free foods and drinks. The benefits to oral health of such policies are potentially great. This style of working is being actively supported by WHO through initiatives such as the Health Promoting Schools Programme (WHO 1997).

> ### DISCUSSION POINTS
>
> The frequent consumption of NMES is the principal cause of dental caries. Use the Ottawa Charter as an outline and devise a range of options that could be adopted to reduce NMES consumption.

DIFFERING APPROACHES TO HEALTH PROMOTION

The practice of health promotion can operate in several different ways, depending upon the philosophy and skills of the practitioner and the setting of the activity.

Five different approaches to health promotion are discussed below to illus-trate the diversity of ways of working within health promotion. Oral health examples will be provided to clarify understanding. The five approaches are:

- preventive;
- behaviour change;
- educational;

- empowerment;
- social change.

Preventive approach

The aim of this approach is a reduction in disease levels, in which medical/dental professionals take the lead. This approach adopts a very *top-down* authoritative style of working, with the health professionals acting as the experts and the patients being passive recipients of preventive care. Interventions such as screening tests or clinical activities such as immunization are used.

Oral health examples could include preventive measures such as fissure sealants or the establishment of a screening programme for oral cancer detection and prevention. One of the major limitations of this style of working is that it does not address the underlying causes of the disease. Therefore new cases will constantly arise and require attention.

Behaviour change

This approach aims to encourage individuals to take responsibility for their health and adopt healthier lifestyles. It is largely based upon the assumption that the provision of information will lead to a sustained change in behaviour. It is an expert-led approach utilizing a range of methods including one-to-one advice and mass media campaigns. The desired changes in lifestyle are determined by the professional and largely imposed on the patient.

Health education advice provided by dentists within surgeries aimed at improving oral hygiene practices is an example of this approach commonly adopted by the dental profession.

Educational approach

To make informed choices about their health-related behaviour, people need not only knowledge but also the skills and attitudes that support this information. The educational approach aims to provide individuals with these. However, unlike the behaviour change approach, it does not set out to persuade a person to change in a particular direction; rather, it is attempting to provide individuals with choices, which they are then able to act upon as they choose.

This approach may use a range of methods to help individuals make an informed choice about their health-related behaviour. In addition to the provision of information, opportunities to explore and share beliefs and attitudes towards health concerns may be very important. Although attitudes may be very difficult to change, having been developed throughout the person's life, group discussions or one-to-one counselling may be useful experiences to enable individuals to explore the basis of their beliefs. Although the educational approach seeks to enhance an individual's overall ability to chose a healthy lifestyle, this approach is still largely led by the expert and ignores the wide range of factors that determine whether an individual has the opportunity or resources to change.

Oral health examples of this approach include school-based educational programmes such as 'Natural Nashers', in which schoolchildren are taught about oral health issues within the curriculum (Craft 1984).

Empowerment

This aims to assist people in identifying their own concerns and priorities, and in developing the confidence and skill to address these issues. Unlike the other approaches, empowerment is essentially a *bottom-up* approach in which the health professional acts as a facilitator. Rather than being the expert, this role involves helping individuals or communities identify their problems and seek appropriate solutions to move things forward. Skills in negotiation, advocacy, and networking are essential requirements for health professionals working in this way.

This approach can be adopted at both an individual and population level. Within clinical settings non-directive counselling techniques can be used to increase people's control over their own lives, although this technique is infrequently used in clinical dentistry. At a population level, community development is a way of empowering groups to become more actively engaged in improving their health and well-being.

Social change

This approach acknowledges the importance of socio-economic and environmental factors in determining health. It therefore aims at changing the physical, social, and economic environments to promote health and well-being. To achieve this requires changes in policy, and political support. Lobbying and policy planning are key elements.

Many health professionals often feel uncomfortable working in such a political arena, but influencing policy-makers at an international, national, or local level is essential to secure good health. For example, in oral health, water fluoridation is largely a political issue which requires political action for its implementation. Only by working closely in a skilful manner with local government and national politicians will progress with this proven public health measure be secured (Evans and Lowry 1999).

WHAT IS THE BEST APPROACH?

Each of the approaches described has certain strengths and weaknesses, so a combination of approaches is probably the best way to promote oral

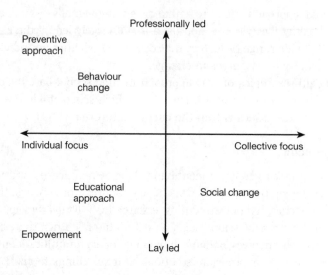

Fig. 9.3 Approaches to health promotion.

health. Clinical dentistry has mainly focused upon the preventive and behaviour change approaches although, as will be discussed later in this chapter, the effectiveness of this style of working has not been demonstrated. Based upon Beattie's (1991) typology, figure 9.3 presents a useful framework for analysing health promotion approaches.

SETTINGS OF HEALTH PROMOTION

Recognition of the importance of the environment on health has led many people working in health promotion to adopt a settings approach to their work. This style of working focuses action upon key settings most influential to health. Table 9.1 presents a range of settings and complementary actions relevant to the promotion of oral health.

DISCUSSION POINTS

Using the example of oral cancer, provide examples of health promotion action across the settings listed in Table 9.1.

EVIDENCE-BASED HEALTH PROMOTION

Within the health service there is an increasing need to demonstrate that interventions are effective at meeting their set objectives and that they contribute to improved health outcomes. This pressure applies equally to both health promotion and treatment interventions. (Details of evidence-based dentistry are provided in Chapter 7.)

Table 9.1 Potential settings, target groups, and activities for oral health promotion

Activity	Settings					Target group					
	Community	Education	Primary Care	Regional	Workplace & national projects	Pre-school	Young	Adults people	Older	Disabled people	Professional groups
Education											
Legislation											
Regulation											
Fiscal											
Organizational change											
Community development											
Reorientation of NHS											

From Daly and Fuller 1996.

In recent years several effectiveness reviews have been undertaken to assess the quality and effect of oral health promotion interventions (Brown 1994; Kay and Locker 1996, 1998; Schou and Locker 1994; Sprod *et al.* 1996). In broad terms, they have all have adopted a similar review method: a systematic search of the published and unpublished oral health promotion literature to determine the overall impact of interventions on a range of outcomes. The common findings of these reviews are shown in Box 9.2.

Publication of these reviews has initiated a lively debate over the future development of oral health promotion services within the NHS. Many experts in health promotion have advocated a cautious interpretation of the findings of effectiveness reviews (Health Education Board for Scotland (HEBS) 1996; Speller *et al.* 1997). It has been argued that the methods employed in the published effectiveness reviews are not appropriate for assessing contemporary health promotion interventions. In Chapter 11 details are given of evaluation methods and measures appropriate for assessing the effects of oral health promotion.

HEALTH PROMOTION STRATEGIES

All over the world many governments have published public health strategies to guide health policy and focus action on improving their populations' health. In the UK, the health departments in Scotland, Wales, England, and Northern Ireland have all recently published strategic frameworks for public health action (visit the Department of Health website for further details: www.doh.gov.uk).

A range of national oral health strategies have also been published in recent years. These documents aim to provide a strategic framework for action to improve oral health in each country. (visit the Department of Health website for further details: www.doh.gov.uk). National oral health targets have been set and broad recommendations for action outlined. However, the success of national strategies is largely dependent upon the development of effective action at a local level. Each local district health authority/board is therefore required to publish a detailed local oral health strategy which translates the national agenda into local action. In 2000 a new NHS Dental Strategy was published, details of which are provided in Chapters 18, 19, 21.

CONCLUSION

Treatment services alone will never successfully alleviate the causes of dental diseases. Health promotion offers the potential to tackle the underlying determinants of oral health and thereby improve the oral health of all sections in society. It involves a range of different strategies, one of which may include health education. The success of health promotion largely depends upon developing partnerships across agencies and, most importantly, actively involving local people in the whole process of health promotion.

Box 9.2 Common findings of oral health promotion effectiveness reviews

The design of studies and the method of evaluation
- Many studies were poorly designed e.g. no control groups used
- Limited evaluation used in most studies
- Evaluation measures when used were of limited value, were not comparable and used inadequate timescales to assess change
- Very basic data analysis undertaken
- Limited reference to contemporary theoretical base

Effectiveness of oral health promotion interventions
- Fluoride remains an effective caries preventive agent
- An individual's knowledge of oral health can be achieved through oral health promotion but the long term impact of this is not clear
- Information alone does not produce long term behaviour changes
- Short term changes in plaque levels can be achieved through oral health promotion interventions. These changes are not sustained over time
- Very few well designed studies have assessed the effectiveness of interventions aiming to reduce sugar consumption.
- In general, cost effectiveness has not been assessed in oral health promotion interventions
- General awareness can be raised by mass media campaigns but they are not effective at promoting knowledge and behaviour change
- There is little evidence for the effectiveness of screening for the early detection of oral cancers

(Watt et al. 2001)

REFERENCES

Beattie, A. (1991). Knowledge and control in health promotion: a test case for social policy and social theory. In *The sociology of the health service* (ed. J. Gabe, M. Calan, and M. Bury), pp. 162–202. London, Routledge.

Blinkhorn, A. (1998). Dental health education: what lessons have we ignored. *British Dental Journal*, **184**, 58–9.

Brown, L. (1994). Research in dental health education and health promotion: a review of the literature. *Health Education Quarterly*, **21**, 83–102.

Craft, M. (1984). Natural Nashers: a programme of dental health education for adolescents in schools. *International Dental Journal*, **34**, 204–13.

Daly, B. and Fuller, S. (1996). *Strengthening oral health promotion in the commissioning process*. Published on behalf of the Oral Health Promotion Research Group. Waterfoot, Lancashire, Eden Bianchi Press.

Evans, D. and Lowry, R. (1999). The privatized water industry and dental public health: water fluoridation. *Community Dental Health*, **16**, 65–6.

Fiske, J., Davis, D., and Horrocks, P. (1995). A self help group for complete denture wearers. *British Dental Journal*, **178**, 18–22.

Kay, L. and Locker, D. (1996). Is dental health education effective? A systematic review of current evidence. *Community Dentistry and Oral Epidemiology*, **24**, 231–5.

Kay, L. and Locker, D. (1998). *A systematic review of the effectiveness of health promotion aimed at promoting oral health.* London, Health Education Authority.

Lalonde, M. (1974). *A new perspective on the health of Canadians.* Ottawa, Health and Welfare Canada.

McGlone, P., Dobson, B., Dowler, E., and Nelson, M. (1999). *Food projects and how they work.* York, York Printing Services.

McKinlay, J. (1979). A case for refocusing upstream: the political economy of health. In *Patients, physicians and illness* (ed. E. Jaco), pp. 96–120. Basingstoke, Macmillan.

Marsh, A. and McKay, S. (1994). *Poor smokers.* London, Policy Studies Institute.

Milio, N. (1986). *Promoting health through public policy.* Ottawa, Canadian Public Health Association.

Health Education Board for Scotland, Research and Evaluation Division (1996). How effective are effectiveness reviews? *Health Education Journal,* **55,** 359–62.

Schou, L. and Locker, D. (1994). *Oral health: a review of the effectiveness of health education and health promotion.* Amsterdam, Dutch Centre for Health promotion and Health Education.

Sheiham, A. and Watt, R. G. (2000). The common risk factor approach: a rational means of promoting oral health. *Community Dentistry and Oral Epidemiology,* **28,** 399–406.

Speller, V., Learmonth, A., and Harrison, D. (1997). The search for evidence of effective health promotion. *British Medical Journal,* **315,** 361–3.

Sprod, A., Anderson, R., and Treasure, E. (1996). *Effective oral health promotion.* [*Literature review.*] Cardiff, Health Promotion Wales.

Watt, R. and Fuller, S. (1999). Oral health promotion – opportunity knocks! *British Dental Journal,* **186,** 3–6.

Watt, R., Fuller, S., Harnett, R., *et al.* (2001). Oral health promotion evaluation – time for development. *Community Dentistry and Oral Epidemiology,* **29,** 161–6.

WHO (World Health Organization) (1984). *Health promotion: a discussion document on the concept and principles.* Copenhagen, WHO.

WHO (World Health Organization) (1986). *The Ottawa Charter for Health Promotion.* Health Promotion 1. iii–v. Geneva, WHO.

WHO (World Health Organization) (1997). *The European Network of health promoting schools.* Copenhagen, WHO.

FURTHER READING

Ewles, L. and Simnett, I. (1999). *Promoting health: a practical guide.* Edinburgh, Baillière Tindall.

Naidoo, J. and Wills, J. (2000). *Health promotion: foundations for practice.* Edinburgh, Baillière Tindall.

Pine, C. (1997). *Community oral health.* Oxford, Wright.

Schou, L. and Blinkhorn, A. (1993). *Oral health promotion.* Oxford, Oxford University Press.

10 Overview of behaviour change

CONTENTS

By the end of this chapter you should be able to:

- Outline the importance of the concepts of behaviour change to dental practice.
- Describe the main elements of a selection of important theories of change.
- Reflect upon personal experiences of attempts at behaviour change and identify important lessons for application in the clinical setting.

This chapter links with:

- Principles of oral health promotion and dental health education (Chapters 9 and X).
- Prevention in practice: caries, periodontal disease, oral cancer, and trauma (Chapters 12–16).

INTRODUCTION

Many dental practitioners become very frustrated with their clients when they fail to follow advice given to improve their oral health. This failure can often be interpreted by dentists as a sign of disinterest, lack of motivation, or sometimes even stupidity! Such an approach helps no one. As has already been identified, to successfully promote oral health the dental team need to work with their clients in a number of ways. For example, to help them select a healthy diet, maintain good oral hygiene, or stop smoking, the dental team need to understand what factors influence these behaviours and how they can be altered successfully.

This chapter therefore aims to review behaviour change to help you understand more fully how you as a clinician can help your clients successfully alter their behaviour to promote and maintain their oral health. Theories and models of behaviour change will be reviewed and consideration will also focus on the practical factors influencing the process of change.

BACKGROUND

Before reviewing the theoretical detail of behaviour change it is important to restate a core principle of public health, that is, the importance of the underlying determinants of health. A wealth of evidence has highlighted that individual behaviours have a relatively limited influence on health outcomes compared to economic, environmental, and social factors (Bartley *et al.* 1997; McKeown 1976; Marmot and Wilkinson 1999; Wilkinson 1996). Therefore any exploration of individual behaviour change needs to take into account the influence of these factors operating at a macro level. However, for health professionals working with individual clients, helping people change their behaviour is an important task within their clinical practice.

Traditionally health professionals have focused largely upon giving their clients information in an attempt to change their behaviour. Such an approach has, however, been mostly unsuccessful at securing long-term changes in behaviour (Sprod *et al.* 1996).

> **DISCUSSION POINTS**
>
> Explain why providing only information to clients may not be successful in changing their behaviour.

Educational theory has identified that there are three domains of learning:
- cognitive;
- affective;
- behavioural.

The cognitive domain refers to the acquisition of factual knowledge and intellectual understanding of ideas. The affective domain is concerned with attitudes, beliefs, and values, whereas the behavioural refers to skills or actions performed. Traditional dental health education was based upon the theory that acquiring new knowledge would alter attitudes and lead to a change in behaviour, the so-called KAB model.

K => A => B

This somewhat simplistic representation of human behaviour rarely exists in the real world. In reality a very complex and dynamic relationship operates between the three domains of learning. In addition, as has been highlighted in Chapter 2, behaviour is largely determined by the opportunities and conditions in which individuals are placed (Sheiham 2000).

THEORIES OF CHANGE

An extensive range of models and theories have been proposed to explain behaviour change. Most have been developed by health psychologists who focus at an individual level and largely ignore the social context within which behaviour is enacted. This section, however, will describe a selection of the more interesting and innovative theories that provide some helpful insights for health professionals seeking to modify their clients' health behaviours.

To help focus your thoughts before reading the theory behind this topic, it would be helpful to reflect upon your own personal experience of changing a behaviour.

DISCUSSION POINTS

Think of an occasion when you have tried to change a certain behaviour, for example eating, smoking, or exercise, and now answer the following questions.

1. What exactly did you try to change?
2. Why did you want to change?
3. What influenced your attempt at a change?
4. Describe what happened when you tried to change?
5. Were you successful with your desired change?
6. What factors made the change more difficult?

Health locus of control (HLOC)

This concept was developed from social-learning theory (Rotter *et al.* 1972) and measures the extent to which individuals believe that their health is influenced either by their own behaviour or by external causes. It is not a measure of actual control of behaviour but rather perceived control over outcomes. Research indicates that the concept is multi-dimensional (Wallston *et al.* 1978). The first dimension is called 'internal HLOC', which represents a person's belief about the impact of their own actions on health outcomes. The other two dimensions refer to external influences on outcomes. 'Powerful others HLOC' focuses on beliefs about the influence of important people on outcomes, whereas 'chance HLOC' refers to the effect of chance or fate on outcomes.

Below are examples illustrating this concept, with reference to periodontal disease.

1. A person with a high internal HLOC would believe that their periodontal health is largely determined by their own ability and skill to effectively remove plaque.
2. Someone with high powerful others HLOC would believe that to maintain their periodontal health, dentists and hygienists are important. These people would therefore believe regular visits to dentists are important for the prevention of periodontal disease.
3. People who score high on chance HLOC would be likely to believe that their periodontal health was determined by chance, and that they could do little to influence the disease process.

Health belief model (HBM)

The health belief model (Becker 1974; Rosenstock 1966) is one of the best known models which explores the function of beliefs in decision-making. The model has been extensively used to predict certain health behaviours but with only limited success in relation to oral health (Søgaard 1993).

Essentially the HBM proposes that when an individual considers changing their behaviour they engage in a cost/benefit analysis of the situation (Fig. 10.1). This would include an assessment of:

- their susceptibility to the health threat;
- the perceived severity of that threat;
- the perceived value of changing the behaviour in question.

In addition, the HBM suggests that before a change of behaviour takes place there needs to be a cue or trigger to initiate an alteration in behaviour. Cues to action may include a range of events such as a comment from a trusted friend, a piece of information on the television, or advice from a dentist.

The concept of self-efficacy has also been included in the model, which stresses that an individual must feel confident and capable of making the desired change in behaviour (Bandura 1977). Without this people do not change successfully.

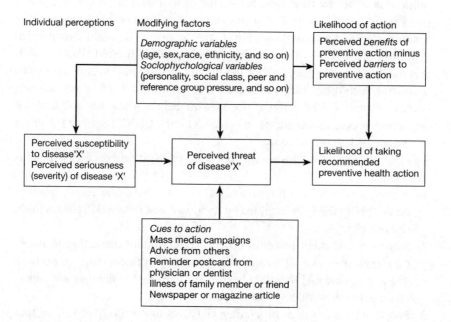

Fig. 10.1 The health belief model. (Reproduced with permission from Sogaard 1993. See Permissions.)

Communication of innovation model

This model, developed originally by Rogers and Shoemaker (1971), explores the process of change at a population level. The theory explains how population groups come to change customary practices and adopt new behaviours. The theory is based upon research in anthropology, sociology, education, communication, and marketing theory and can be applied to a variety of target populations including professional groups.

Different categories of adopters are identified dependent upon individuals' awareness and willingness to try out new practices (Fig. 10.2). For example, *innovators* are individuals eager to experiment with new behaviours. They tend to be middle-class people who are adventurous and keen to find out information about new ideas, mostly from the media. They are closely followed by *early adopters*, who tend to be respected members of society. In turn they are succeeded by the *early majority*, who adopt new ideas deliberately just ahead of Mr/Ms. Average. These first three groups all make the decision to change based upon a reasoned analysis of the costs and benefits of an innovation. The penultimate group are the *late majority*, who are usually lower in social standing and learn new ideas from peers through established social networks. *Laggards*, the last group to adopt an innovation, tend to be socially isolated and unresponsive to new ideas and social pressures. When the proportion of those who adopt the innovation is plotted against time, a characteristically S-shaped curve results.

Although developed over 25 years ago, this theory clearly still has direct relevance to health promotion practice. For example, the processes of adoption of change within populations could help in the development of interventions designed to tackle health inequalities through targeting defined subgroups. The influence of certain sections of the middle class as early adopters should not be overlooked; they can be very valuable as opinion leaders and agents of change within the wider society.

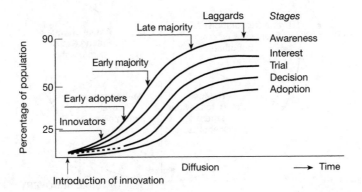

Fig. 10.2 Diffusion of innovation. (Reproduced with permission from Sogaard 1993. See Permissions.)

Stages of change model

This model was developed by a US research team originally investigating the processes involved in smoking cessation (Prochaska and DiClemente 1983). The model has since been revised and applied to a whole range of health-related behaviours including diet change, exercise, and drug use. Recently a range of health education materials based around the model have been developed for use in primary care settings.

The model is based on the assumption that behaviour change is a dynamic, non-linear process that involves several distinct stages (Fig. 10.3). At the *precontemplation* stage an individual has not even considered changing his or her behaviour, whereas in *contemplation* a person is thinking over the pros and cons of making a change. *Preparation* is the stage when a person is making definite plans to change, in *action* the actual behaviour change is initiated, and in *maintenance* the modified behaviour is actively sustained. The model recognizes that for many people changing behaviour is a difficult and prolonged process which may involve many attempts, as *relapses* often occur in the process. Marlatt and Gordon (1980) have identified that these relapses are most often caused by:

• negative emotional states;
• interpersonal conflict;
• social pressures.

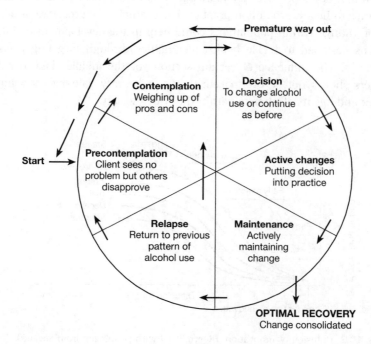

Fig. 10.3 Stages of change model

DISCUSSION POINTS

The stages of change model identifies different points in the process of change. Identify how dental professionals could help their patients successfully modify their tooth-brushing behaviour. Consider what could be done at each stage in the model.

Although this model has been criticized as an over-simplistic representation of change, it does provide insights into the processes involved when an individual changes certain behaviours. Of particular importance is the need to target varied interventions to people who are at the different stages of change and not to assume everyone is ready or willing to change (Campbell *et al.* 1994). It is also important to recognize the routine nature of relapsing, and the need for health professionals to provide support and encouragement at this crucial point in the process.

Life course analysis

This theory is based upon an analysis of the complex ways in which biological risk interacts with economic, social, and psychological factors in the development of chronic disease throughout the entire course of life (Bartley *et al.* 1997; Kuh and Ben Shlomo 1997). For example, epidemiological evidence from cohort studies which have closely monitored the health and development of groups of people, beginning at birth and continuing throughout adulthood, have demonstrated the long-term effects of low birth weight. When very small babies reach adulthood, they have a far greater chance of experiencing a range of chronic conditions such as heart disease (Barker 1994).

In the life course perspective particular emphasis is placed on the social context, and the interaction between people and their environments in the passage through life. This approach is of value in assessing how advantage and disadvantage may cluster at *socially critical periods* of social development and accumulate longitudinally. For example, a child born into a very poor family may suffer the consequences of growing up in an unhealthy environment. Serious accidents during childhood may occur which could affect schooling and educational achievement. A lack of qualifications limits access to higher education and then the prospects of getting a good job are greatly reduced. During childhood and adolescence a poor diet, smoking, and limited exercise all contribute to a greater risk of disease in adulthood. A spiral of events and circumstances collectively affect the well-being and health of the individual throughout his or her life.

Box 10.1 presents a range of critical periods in human development that may have particular importance in determining health status and the generation of health inequalities within populations.

In relation to oral health there is good evidence that stressful life events such as divorce can have a detrimental impact on periodontal health

> **Box 10.1** Critical periods in human development most relevant to health
>
> 1. Transition from primary to secondary school.
> 2. School examinations.
> 3. Entry to labour market.
> 4. Leaving parental home.
> 5. Establishing own residence.
> 6. Transition to parenthood.
> 7. Job insecurity, change, or loss.
> 8. Exit from labour market.
>
> *(Bartley* et al. *1997)*

(Croucher *et al.* 1997). The insights provided from this theoretical perspective may have implications for the timing and nature of health, social, and welfare support, particularly in relation to tackling health inequalities and supporting and protecting vulnerable groups in society.

Social capital

Social capital is a relatively recent theory that has provoked a great deal of interest and debate from many people working in public health research and policy. It is defined as *'features of social organisation, such as civic participation, norms of reciprocity, and trust in others, that facilitate co-operation for mutual benefit'* (Putnam 1993). The theory of social capital has been developed from a political science analysis of the functions of local government in Italy. It is essentially assessing the level of social trust that operates within a community, how safe people feel together, how much help people give each other for their own and collective benefit, and the degree of involvement in social and community issues such as voting and community groups.

A research group from the Harvard School of Public Health has recently published results from a study in which data from the US General Social Survey was assessed to measure the relationship between measures of social capital, income inequality, and mortality in 39 states across the US (Kawachi *et al.* 1997). The results indicated that income inequality was strongly associated with lack of social trust and that states with high levels of social mistrust had higher age-adjusted mortality rates from a range of conditions, including coronary heart disease, malignant neoplasms, cerebrovascular disease, unintentional injury, and infant mortality.

To date very little research has assessed the relationship between oral health and social capital, but when one considers the common risks of diet, smoking, and accidents associated with heart disease, cancers, trauma, and dental diseases, a strong relationship may well exist between oral health and certain elements of social capital. A recent study in Brazil has demonstrated an inverse relationship between the percentage of caries free children and measures of social cohesion (Patussi *et al.* 2001).

Kawachi and colleagues concluded that 'the growing gap between the rich and the poor affects the social organisation of communities and that the resulting damage to the social fabric may have profound implications for the public's health.'

The implications for public health of the theory of social capital and social cohesion are potentially profound. What role do health workers have in facilitating improved social networks, social support, and community involvement? Community development approaches within health promotion clearly fit very well into this agenda.

PRACTICAL REFLECTIONS ON THEORIES OF BEHAVIOUR CHANGE

The theoretical research into behaviour change reviewed above may appear very abstract and detached from the realities of clinical dental practice. However, there are certain important issues of relevance that should be highlighted. This is best achieved by reflecting back upon personal experiences of behaviour change. On p. 157 a series of questions was posed to encourage you to consider your own experience. Think back to your responses to these questions and consider the ideas presented in the theoretical overview.

Process of change

Very rarely do individuals manage to change an established behaviour at one attempt. For most people several attempts are required before they can successfully change a habit. This process may take several months, or even years, and for many people can be seen as a constant battle. A whole host of factors, many of which may be outside the control of the individual, influence progress with desired change.

Motivations to change

When you reviewed your experiences of changing a behaviour it may have become very apparent that the initial motivation for changing was not primarily health reasons. Clinicians often forget that for most ordinary people, teeth and gums are not the single most important issue in their complex lives. Individuals often reduce their sugars intake not due to concerns about their caries risk but because of worries about their weight or body shape (Watt 1997). Even with something as potentially damaging to the health as smoking, people's motivations to quit are often far more complex and diverse. It is therefore important to recognize the varying motivations individuals may have for changing their behaviours. Health-directed behaviour change may be important for people who are especially concerned about their health. For many, however, social, financial, and other practical concerns may be of paramount importance in their motivations to change, with health issues, so-called health-related behaviour change, being of secondary concern.

Barriers preventing change

Most of us, no matter how determined we may be to change, often do not succeed with our attempt. This is principally due to the many barriers (listed in Box 10.2) that prevent us from achieving long-term sustained changes.

Box 10.2 Barriers to achieving long-term change

- Lack of opportunity – for example, limited access to healthier snacks in school tuckshops.
- Lack of resources – for example, unable to afford new toothbrushes for large family.
- Lack of support – for example, living with a smoker when you want to quit.
- Conflicting information on nature of change – for example, confusion over health education messages.
- Conflicting motives – for example, enjoyment associated with eating sugary snacks with friends.
- Long-term nature of benefit – for example, lung cancer doesn't affect teenagers for another 40 years and smoking has immediate personal and social benefits.
- Belief that change not possible – for example, when someone has tried to improve their tooth-brushing technique before without success.
- No clearly defined goals – for example, asking someone to stop eating sugar altogether when so many processed foods have sugars added to them.
- Lack of knowledge on what to change – for example, people's beliefs that fruit juices are full of vitamins so they must be good for their baby.

(Jacob and Plamping 1989)

IMPLICATIONS FOR CLINICAL PRACTICE AND HEALTH PROMOTION

Key implications of behaviour change

What implications can be drawn from this exploration of behaviour change? Well, there are several fundamental lessons that can be highlighted:

Importance of context and environment

Individual behaviours are largely determined by complex array of factors beyond the control of most individuals. 'Victim blaming' helps no one, least of all individuals with the greatest oral health needs.

Limitations of information alone

Leaflets, posters, videos, and websites which concentrate on imparting oral health knowledge will only be of limited value to most people. Behaviour change is complex and most people are well-informed about the basic oral health messages.

Process of change

Most people will have extensive experience of attempting to change their eating patterns or quitting smoking, the so-called health career. It is essential to take a detailed history of a person's previous experiences of change and learn from this. Target interventions to match individuals' desire and abilities to change.

Support essential

If you have struggled to change elements of your behaviour, be understanding and supportive with others in your clinical environment. Encouragement, understanding, and empathy are all essential to enable your clients achieve their goals.

CONCLUSION

This chapter has introduced some of the key theory and practical issues relevant to understanding behaviour change. To be a successful clinician you will need to be able to influence your clients and assist them with desired changes. Success in helping clients to alter their behaviours will largely depend upon your awareness of the factors and processes influencing behaviour change. The provision of information alone in most cases will be insufficient to achieve sustained changes in behaviour to promote oral health.

REFERENCES

Bandura, A. (1977). *Social learning theory*. London, Prentice Hall.

Barker, D. (1994). *Mothers, babies and disease in later life*. London, British Medical Journal Publishing.

Bartley, M., Blane, D., and Montgomery, S. (1997) Socio-economic determinants of health; health and the life course: why safety nets matter. *British Medical Journal*, **314**, 1194–6.

Becker, M. (1974). The health belief model and personal health behaviour. *Health Education Monographs*, **2**, 1–146.

Campbell, M. DeVellis, B., Strecher, V. *et al.* (1994). Improving dietary behaviour: the effectiveness of tailored messages in primary care settings. *Journal of Public Health*, **84**, 783–7.

Croucher, R., Torres, M., Hughes, F., and Sheiham, A. (1997). The relationship between life events and periodontitis: a case control study. *Clinical Periodontology*, **24**, 39–43.

Jacob, M. and Plamping, D. (1989). *The practice of primary dental care.* London, Wright.

Kawachi, I., Kennedy, B. P., Lochner, K., and Prothrow-Stith, D. (1997) Social capital, income inequality and mortality. *American Journal of Public Health*, **87**, 1491–8.

Kuh, D. and Ben Shlomo, Y. (ed.) (1997). *A life course approach to adult disease.* Oxford University Press.

McKeown, T. (1976). *The role of medicine: dream, mirage or nemesis?* London, Nuffield Provincial Hospital Trust.

Marlatt, G. and Gordon, J. (1980). Determinants of relapse: implications for the maintenance of behaviour change. In *Behavioural medicine: changing health lifestyles* (ed. P. Davidson and S. Davidson), pp. 291–341. New York, Brunner/Mazel.

Marmot, M. and Wilkinson, R. G. (ed.) (1999). *Social determinants of health.* Oxford, Oxford University Press.

Patussi, M., Marcenes, W., Croucher, R., and Sheiham, A. (2001). The relationship between dental caries in 6 to 12 year old Brazilian school children and social deprivation, income inequality and social cohesion. *Social Science and Medicine.* (In press.)

Prochaska, J. and DiClemente, C. (1983). Stages and processes of self change in smoking: toward an integrative model of change. *Journal of Consulting and Clinical Psychology*, **51**, 390–5.

Putnam, R. (1993) *Making democracy work.* Princeton University Press.

Rogers, E. and Shoemaker, F. (1971). *Communication of innovations: a cross-cultural approach.* New York, Free Press.

Rosenstock, I. (1966). Why people use health services. *Millbank Memorial Fund Quarterly*, **44**, 94–121.

Rotter, J., Chance, J., and Phares, E. (1972). *Applications of a social-learning theory.* New York, Holt, Rinehart and Winston.

Sheiham, A. (2000). Improving oral health for all: focusing on determinants and conditions. *Health Education Journal*, **59**, 64–76.

Søgaard, A. (1993). Theories and models of health behaviour. In *Oral health promotion* (ed. L. Schou and A. Blinkhorn), pp. 25–64. Oxford, Oxford University Press.

Sprod, A., Anderson, R., and Treasure, E. (1996). *Effective oral health promotion.* [*Literature review.*] Cardiff, Health Promotion Wales.

Wallston, K., Wallston, B., and DeVillis, R. (1978). Development of the multi-dimensional health locus of control scales. *Health Education Monographs*, **6**, 160–70.

Watt, R. G. (1997). Stages of change for sugar and fat reduction in an adolescent sample. *Community Dental Health*, **14**, 102–8.

Wilkinson, R. G. (1996) *Unhealthy societies.* London, Routledge.

FURTHER READING

Søgaard, A. (1993). Theories and models of health behaviour. In *Oral health promotion* (ed. L. Schou and A. Blinkhorn), pp. 25–64. Oxford, Oxford University Press.

11 Oral health education in dental practice settings

CONTENTS

By the end of this chapter you should be able to:

- Define health education.
- Outline the key messages in oral health education.
- Describe the steps involved in planning health education.
- Present an overview of the different methods and materials used in health education.
- Outline the principles of evaluation of health education.

This chapter links with:
- Principles of oral health promotion (Chapter 9).
- Overview of behaviour change (Chapter 10).
- Prevention of caries, periodontal disease, oral cancer, and dental trauma (Chapters 12–16).

INTRODUCTION

As outlined in Chapter 9, in recent years a range of national oral health strategies have been published, all of which have stressed the important role dental professionals have to play in promoting oral health through health education (Department of Health 2000). Effectiveness reviews of oral health education have, however, questioned the long-term value of many health education programmes in achieving sustained improvements in oral health (Brown 1994; Kay and Locker 1996; Schou and Locker 1994; Sprod *et al.* 1996). It is therefore important that dental health professionals understand the principles of health education and the most effective ways of delivering it within clinical settings.

DEFINITION OF HEALTH EDUCATION

Health education is defined as any educational activity which aims to achieve a health-related goal (WHO 1984). Activity can be directed at individuals, groups, or even populations. There are three main domains of learning (see also Chapter 10):

- **Cognitive**: understanding factual knowledge (for example, knowledge that eating sugary snacks is linked to the development of dental decay).
- **Affective**: emotions, feelings, and beliefs associated with health (for example, belief that baby teeth are not important).

- **Behavioural**: skills development (for example, skills required to effectively floss teeth).

DISCUSSION POINTS

Traditionally health education was confined to schools and concentrated largely on increasing students' knowledge of various health issues.
What are the limitations of this approach?
Why was this the dominant approach in health education for so long?
What alternative approach for oral health education would you recommend?

How do knowledge, attitudes, and behaviours relate to each other? For most people, in most instances, the relationship is complex, dynamic, and very personal; very rarely is it linear. In other words, human beings are not purely rational in their thoughts, feelings, and actions. For example, the vast majority of smokers are fully aware that smoking is a major risk factor for lung cancers and a whole host of other conditions. This knowledge, however, does not stop them smoking. When knowledge conflicts with behaviour, it is known as cognitive dissonance. Many smokers believe the habit is dirty and socially unattractive, but such attitudes do not stop people from smoking.

Later in this chapter the different methods that can be used to address the domains of learning will be explored. With such a complex and dynamic relationship existing between knowledge, attitudes, and behaviour, it is essential that all three elements are appropriately covered in health education.

Chapter 9 outlined that health education is one of the strategies within a health promotion policy. Health education and health promotion are therefore not the same thing, and the two terms should be used carefully, as appropriate.

THE SCIENTIFIC BASIS OF ORAL HEALTH EDUCATION

It is very important that the health education messages given to the public are consistent and scientifically correct. The public are increasingly sceptical of health information, and many people believe that experts disagree on what health advice to follow (Sheiham *et al.* 1990). This confusion is no accident: it is purposively created by vested interest groups who deliberately attempt to confuse the public to lessen the impact and credibility of health messages.

In an attempt to clarify the core oral health education messages, the Health Education Authority published a consensus document (Levine 1996). This was produced by a group of leading figures in the oral health sciences, and is a distillation of published evidence on effective preventive strategies.

The key messages are:

- **Diet**: reduce the consumption, and especially frequency of intake, of food and drinks containing sugar (NMES).
- **Tooth-brushing**: clean the teeth thoroughly twice every day with a fluoride toothpaste.
- **Dental attendance**: visit a dentist once a year for an oral examination.
- **Fluoridation**: request the local water company to supply water with the optimum fluoride level (0.7–1.0 ppm).

PLANNING ORAL HEALTH EDUCATION

To be effective health education needs to be properly planned and organized (Watt and Fuller 1999). Planning provides a clear defined structure to an activity, focuses action on the needs of the target group, and avoids duplication of activity. It also ensures that activity is fully evaluated to inform a review process when any lessons can be learned for future action.

Many different approaches to planning have been proposed. In this chapter two well-known planning models will be presented, and oral health examples will be used to illustrate their value.

Health education planning model

This a very popular practical model designed by Ewles and Simnett (1999), which provides a step-by-step guide to planning health education. It can be used in planning activity on a one-to-one basis or for groups (Fig. 11.1). To illustrate the value of the model an example of clinical oral health education will be used.

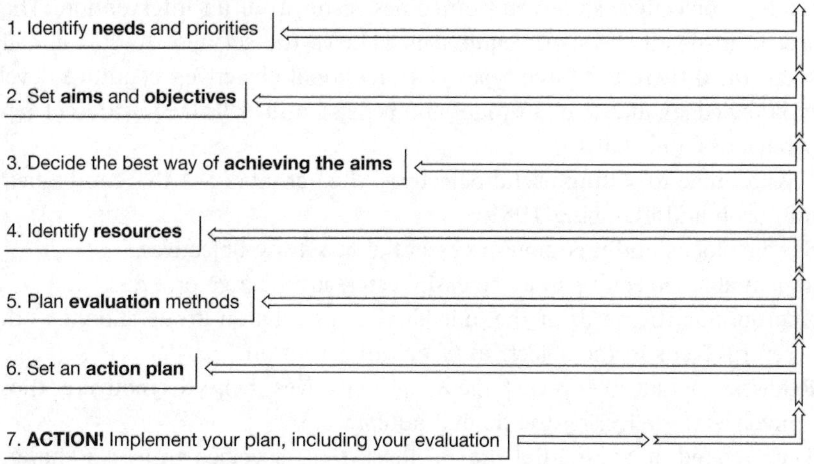

1. Identify **needs** and priorities
2. Set **aims** and **objectives**
3. Decide the best way of **achieving the aims**
4. Identify **resources**
5. Plan **evaluation** methods
6. Set an **action plan**
7. **ACTION!** Implement your plan, including your evaluation

Fig. 11.1 A flowchart for planning and evaluating health education. (Reproduced from Ewles and Simnett 1999 with permission from Harcourt Publishers Ltd. See Permissions.)

Identify client and their characteristics

Within a dental practice a wide range of different people may be identified as requiring oral health education. However, it is important to select specific groups to ensure activity is tailored to their particular needs. For this example an adolescent client who is undergoing orthodontic treatment will be the identified client.

Identify client needs

It is essential that the needs of the client are clearly and fully identified before any action is undertaken. Traditionally client needs have been assessed exclusively by the dentist based upon clinical data only (normative need). Such an approach has many limitations (see Chapter 3 for a full discussion of the concepts of need). In planning effective health education both professionally defined need and the client's concerns (felt and expressed need) have to be taken into consideration. In this example, the clinical data might indicate a problem with plaque accumulation and gingivitis in relation to a fixed appliance. The client, however, might be more concerned about the appearance of bleeding gums and his/her bad breath.

Decide aims for health education

Based upon the assessed needs of the client an aim can be set, specifying the desired change that is planned. One aim in this oral health example could be to improve and maintain the client's periodontal health through more effective plaque control. This aim indicates what change is desired and is relevant to the defined needs of the client.

Formulate specific objectives

Goals or objectives state what outcomes result from an intervention. They specify in detail the steps required to achieve the set aim. As has already been stated there are three types of educational objectives: cognitive (levels of knowledge), affective (attitudes and beliefs), and skills (acquisition of new behaviours and skills).

As a guide to setting useful objectives, the acronym SMART can be helpful (Jacob and Plamping 1989):

Specific: focus and precision are essential in setting objectives.

Measurable: objectives must be easily assessed to gauge progress.

Appropriate: the needs of the individual or population group should be the central focus in the objectives of any intervention.

Realistic: achievable yet challenging objectives help to motivate those involved in delivering the desired outcomes.

Time related: it is essential that a timescale is specified to assess changes achieved.

A SMART objective could be: within 4 weeks the patient will reduce gingival swelling through twice-daily tooth-brushing.

Identify resources

Once the desired aim and objectives have been decided and agreed, the resources available to implement the intervention need to be identified. In health education, resources may include people's expertise and existing skill, and materials such as leaflets or oral hygiene aids.

Plan content and method in detail

By this stage the content and method of the intervention should be apparent. To teach an adolescent improved oral hygiene skills would require several different components. Merely handing out a leaflet is not sufficient to improve a complex and manually challenging activity such as effective tooth-brushing. Such a skill-based activity requires a demonstration, an opportunity for practise and, most importantly, constructive feedback.

Plan evaluation methods

A full evaluation of any health education intervention is a very important element that is often forgotten. Evaluation is designed to assess whether the set aim and goals have been achieved, so evaluation measures that are appropriate to these must be selected. In relation to tooth-brushing a range of evaluation measures could be chosen: these might include plaque scores, tooth-brushing frequency, or even certain knowledge-based measures. A more detailed account of evaluation will be provided in Part x.

Action: carry out activity

At last it is time to get on with the planned intervention!

Evaluate

Evaluation information can be collected both during and at the end of the intervention to assess the impact of the activity.

Review

Once all the steps have been completed it is useful to review the whole process to draw out useful lessons for future use. Practice makes perfect.

PRECEDE model of health education

The PRECEDE (Predisposing, Reinforcing, and Enabling Causes in Educational Diagnosis and Evaluation) is a planning model that provides a structure for the different steps involved in designing a behaviour change intervention (Fig. 11.2) (Green *et al.* 1980).

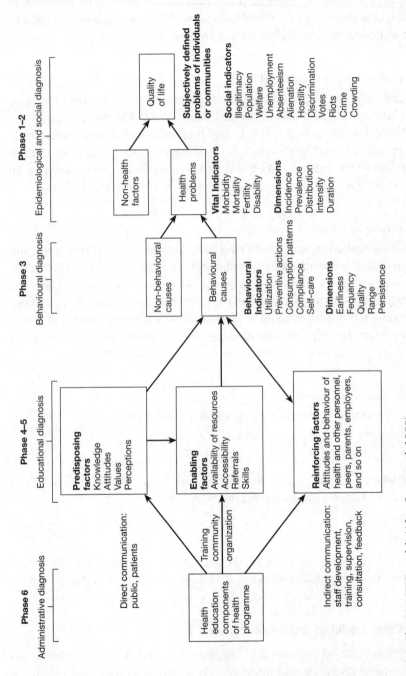

Fig. 11.2 The PRECEDE model. (After Green *et al.* 1980)

As presented in Fig. 11.2, the model is composed of the following key phases.

Phases 1–2: Epidemiological and social diagnoses

Health problems are identified through analysis of epidemiological data and the community's perceptions of need. (Non-health factors are excluded from further consideration as they are deemed outside the remit of health education.)

Phase 3: Behavioural diagnosis

As this model concentrates upon planning interventions to promote behavioural change, non-behavioural causes of health problems, such as poverty and unhealthy environments, are excluded from further investigation. Instead the behavioural causes are identified and ranked in importance before proceeding to the next phase.

Phases 4–5: Educational diagnosis

Three categories of factors affecting behaviour are then identified and analysed to select the most important factors to focus upon in the intervention. Predisposing factors, such as a person's knowledge, values, and perceptions, all affect their motivation to change. Enabling factors are the range of skills and resources required to enact the motivated behaviour, whereas reinforcing factors refer to the feedback received from significant others such as family, friends, or colleagues, which may promote or hinder the process of behaviour change.

Phase 6: Administrative diagnosis

Based upon the findings of the previous phases, the development, implementation, and evaluation of an appropriate health education intervention is then possible.

DISCUSSION POINTS

The PRECEDE model may seem rather complex and confusing at first sight. As an illustration, consider the following example.

As you are a dental practitioner, the local residential care home requests your assistance in providing oral health education for the clients and staff.

1. What oral health problems may be affecting older people living in a residential home?

2. What behaviour changes would improve the oral health of the residents? (Consider both staff and residents.)

3. Describe potential predisposing, enabling, and reinforcing factors affecting oral health behaviours.

4. Outline possible health education interventions appropriate for this example.

HEALTH EDUCATION METHODS AND MATERIALS

A wide variety of health education methods can be used, with the final selection depending upon the aim of the intervention and the most appropriate means of meeting it. Box 11.1 provides an example of the methods that could be used in the promotion of oral health.

Box 11.1 Oral health education methods

- One-to-one supervision
- Group work
- Interactive computer software
- Lectures
- Peer education
- Group discussion
- Role play
- Mass media

A vast array of oral health education materials are produced each year by a wide selection of both commercial and NHS organizations. Box 11.2 lists a range of different types of health education materials. Each of these resources has certain advantages and disadvantages depending on how they are used.

Box 11.2 Health education materials

- Information sheets
- Flipcharts
- Black/whiteboards
- Leaflets
- Posters
- Display boards
- Videos
- Audio cassettes
- Overhead projector transparencies
- Computer programs

It is essential that the best quality and most appropriate materials are used in clinical settings. Box 11.3 presents a set of criteria that can be used to assess the quality of materials, and therefore facilitate the selection of the best.

To facilitate the distribution of high-quality resources, directories of health education resources have been produced (Blinkhorn *et al.* 2000). These catalogues enable practitioners to assess what materials are available and where they can be ordered from.

> **Box 11.3** Quality criteria to assess health education materials
>
> - Funding source: conflicts of interest?
> - Process of development: indications of collaborative working?
> - Objectives: implied or stated?
> - Target audience: is this clearly stated?
> - Scientific content: conforms to Levine (1996) guidelines.
> - Presentation quality: professional presentation; use of appropriate images, layout, and style of text?
> - Appeal: interesting feel, stimulating, engaging?
> - Equal opportunities: consideration given to population diversity?
> - Understandability: use of jargon, chunks of dense text, plain language?
> - Practical focus: application of content?

DISCUSSION POINTS

Critically apply the above criteria to a selection of health education leaflets. What are the main strengths and weaknesses of the materials you have reviewed?

TEAM APPROACH TO ORAL HEALTH EDUCATION

To be effective within clinical dental settings health education needs to be incorporated within the workload of the whole dental team (Sheiham 1992). However, each team member needs to have a clearly defined role and understand the respective responsibilities of their colleagues. Developing health education within dental practices can therefore act as a useful team building exercise.

As the leader and manager of the dental team it is essential that the dentist directs and supports any health education activity. In conjunction with their clinical role, dentists should be involved in assessing their clients' health education needs, and where appropriate providing opportunistic advice and support. When more intensive health education support is required, dentists should then be able to refer these individuals to other members of the team who have the time, resources, and skills required. In addition to these diagnostic and referral functions dentists should also perform a co-ordinating role, overseeing the evaluation and monitoring of health education activity within their practices.

Auxiliary staff involved in health education, such as dental nurses and hygienists, need to have the appropriate training in health education to successfully perform their tasks.

DISCUSSION POINTS

Smoking cessation is an expanding area of health education within many primary care settings.

Within the setting of a dental practice, outline the key roles and responsibilities of the different members of the dental team in smoking cessation.

SKILLS IN ORAL HEALTH EDUCATION

Just as learning how to cut a cavity correctly involves the acquisition of a range of technical and scientific skills, delivering effective health education requires a wide range of skills which take time, practice, and experience to fully develop. Some of these key skills are listed in Box 11.4.

Box 11.4 Health education skills

- Communication skills
    - Appropriate questioning
    - Active listening
    - Summarizing information
    - Giving feedback
- Assessing needs
- Motivational interviewing
- Presentational skills
- Goal-setting
- Teaching skills
- Working with small groups
- Measuring and monitoring change

SETTINGS FOR ORAL HEALTH EDUCATION

Oral health education can take place in a wide variety of settings as shown in Box 11.5. A gradual shift is taking place, away from the traditional schools-based activity to a broader-based approach which targets action at influential decision-makers rather than attempting to educate every school child in an area (upstream approach). This form of health education attempts to focus action on key individuals or organizations who then can cascade the health education advice to a wider audience. Not only is this approach more likely to achieve sustained changes but is also a far more cost-effective way of working.

There are many different important partners to work with in oral health education (Box 11.6). Dentists and their teams working within the

---

Box 11.5 Settings for oral health education

- Primary care
- Hospitals and clinics
- Schools and colleges
- Pre-school education and care
- Local authority services
- Commercial organizations
- Workplace
- Community-based initiatives
- Older people's residential homes

Box 11.6 Potential partners in oral health education

- General practitioners
- Health visitors
- School nurses
- Pharmacists
- Teachers
- School governors
- Pre-school carers
- Local authority staff
- Politicians – local and national government
- Voluntary sector workers
- Media
- Business and commercial people
- Lecturers – FE colleges

General Dental Services may have established links with colleagues in other primary care professions such as GPs, health visitors, and pharmacists. However, there are many groups outside of the health service who may also have an important role in oral health education. The community dental services and/or health promotion departments should have links with these groups.

PRINCIPLES OF EVALUATION

Evaluation should be a core element in the planning of any health service activity, whether it be a treatment or health promotion activity. Evaluation is the process of assessing what has been achieved and how it has been achieved. It is therefore a critical appraisal of any activity to assess what were the good and bad features, and ways of improving future activity. Both outcome and process evaluation measures can be assessed.

Outcome evaluation is designed to assess what has been achieved and whether the objectives set have been reached. A whole range of outcome measures can be used in health promotion evaluation, depending upon the nature of the activity undertaken. For example, outcome measures could include assessing changes in health awareness, knowledge or attitude, or policy (Nutbeam 1998). In some circumstances changes in health status could be used as an outcome measure for certain health education interventions. However, this is only appropriate when the intervention is a long-term programme capable of achieving such a change (Watt *et al.* 2001). A whole range of methods can be used to measure health education outcomes. These include questionnaires, interviews, policy reviews, or health surveys, depending on which outcomes are being assessed.

In health education, in addition to measuring the outcomes it is important to also assess the processes involved in developing and implementing an intervention. Process evaluation therefore aims to assess the quality of the implementation. Were the most appropriate methods and materials used? Was the timescale appropriate? Were resources used efficiently?

DISCUSSION POINTS

Within a dental surgery the staff are planning a health education programme targeted at reducing the sugars consumption of their patients under 5 years old. Suggest what would be some suitable outcome and process evaluation measures for such an intervention.

CONCLUSIONS

Oral health education is an important part of oral health promotion and should be an important part of all dental professionals' clinical duties. Effective oral health education within dental practices is largely dependent upon detailed planning and teamwork. It is important that all health education advice and support is based upon scientifically sound evidence.

REFERENCES

Blinkhorn, A., Blinkhorn, F., Davis, K., and Draper, H. (2000). *Catalogue of dental health resources*. Manchester, Eden Bianchi Press.

Brown, L. (1994). Research in dental health education and health promotion: a review of the literature. *Health Education Quarterly*, **21**, 83–102.

Department of Health (2000). *Modernising NHS dentistry: implementing the NHS plan*. London, Department of Health.

Ewles, L. and Simnett, I. (1999). *Promoting health: a practical guide*. Edinburgh, Baillière Tindall.

Green, L., Kreuter, M., Deeds, S., and Partridge, K. (1980). *Health education planning: a diagnostic approach*. Mountain View, California, USA, Mayfield Publishing.

Jacob, C. and Plamping, D. (1989). *The practice of primary dental care*. London, Wright.

Kay, L. and Locker, D. (1996). Is dental health education effective? A systematic review of current evidence. *Community Dentistry and Oral Epidemiology*, **24**, 231–5.

Levine, R. (1996). *The scientific basis of dental health education: a policy document* (4th edn). London, Health Education Authority.

Nutbeam, D. (1998). Evaluating health promotion: progress, problems and solutions. *Health Promotion International*, **13**, 27–44.

Schou, L. and Blinkhorn, A. (1993). *Oral health promotion*. Oxford, Oxford University Press.

Schou, L. and Locker, D. (1994). *Oral health: a review of the effectiveness of health education and health promotion*. Amsterdam, Dutch Centre for Health promotion and Health Education.

Sheiham, A. (1992). The role of the dental team in promoting dental health and general health through oral health. *International Dental Journal*, **42**, 223–8.

Sheiham, A., Marmot, M., Taylor, B., and Brown, A. (1990). Recipes for health. In *British social attitudes: the 1990/1991 report* (ed. R. Jowell, S. Witherspoon, and L. Brook), pp. 250–68. Aldershot, Gower.

Sprod, A., Anderson, R., and Treasure, E. (1996). *Effective oral health promotion*. [*Literature review.*] Cardiff, Health Promotion Wales.

Watt, R. and Fuller, S. (1999). Oral health promotion: opportunity knocks! *British Dental Journal*, **186**, 3–6.

Watt, R., Fuller, S., Harnett, R., *et al.* (2001). Oral health promotion evaluation: time for development. *Community Dentistry and Oral Epidemiology*, **29**, 161–6.

WHO (World Health Organization) (1984). *Health promotion: a discussion document on the concepts and principles*. Copenhagen, WHO.

FURTHER READING

Ewles, L. and Simnett, I. (1999). *Promoting health: a practical guide*. Edinburgh, Baillière Tindall.

Naidoo, J. and Wills, J. (2000). *Health promotion: foundations for practice*. Edinburgh, Baillière Tindall.

Pine, C. (1997). *Community oral health*. Oxford, Wright.

Schou, L. and Blinkhorn, A. (1993). *Oral health promotion*. Oxford, Oxford University Press.

Sheiham, A. and Croucher, R. (1994). Current perspectives on improving chairside dental health education for adults. *International Dental Journal*, **44**, 202–6.

12 Sugars and caries prevention

CONTENTS

By the end of this chapter you should be able to:

- Present a classification of sugars based upon government recommendations.
- Critically outline the principal sources of evidence on the relationship between sugars consumption and caries development.
- Describe ways of assisting individuals reduce their sugars consumption.
- Outline approaches to reduce sugars consumption at a population level.

This chapter links with:
- Determinants of health (Chapter 2).
- Trends in oral health (Chapter 6).
- Principles of oral health promotion (Chapter 9).
- Overview of behaviour change (Chapter 10).
- Oral health education in dental practice settings (Chapter 11).

INTRODUCTION

Dental caries remains the single most important oral condition treated by the dental profession on a daily basis. From a public health perspective the prevention of caries is still therefore a major challenge. As outlined in Chapter 4, before effective prevention can be delivered the cause of the condition needs to be fully understood. In addition, the disease process should be clear. This chapter will review the evidence on the aetiology of dental caries and present an overview of preventive measures that can be adopted at an individual clinical level, as well as community wide.

CARIES PROCESS

Before reviewing the aetiology of caries it is important to recall the nature of the disease process. A clear understanding of the process of caries is essential for the development of effective preventive strategies.

> ### DISCUSSION POINTS
>
> Based upon your dental sciences and clinical teaching:
> - Describe the key anatomical features of a caries lesion.
> - Review the demineralization and remineralization process within a caries lesion.
> - Identify the range of factors that may inhibit the demineralization and aid the remineralization process.

Caries is a dynamic process involving alternating periods of demineralization and remineralization by acids, mainly from sugars. However, the majority of lesions in permanent teeth advance slowly, with an average lesion taking at least 3 years to progress through enamel to dentine (Mejare *et al.* 1998). In populations with low DMF/dmf levels the majority of carious lesions are confined to the occlusal surfaces of the molar teeth. At higher DMF/dmf levels smooth surfaces may also be affected by caries (McDonald and Sheiham 1992).

SUGARS CLASSIFICATION

Many different terms have been used to name and classify sugars. This has caused a degree of confusion amongst both the general public and health professionals. In recognition of this an expert government committee – Committee on Medical Aspects of Food Policy (COMA) have recommended a revised naming system, which has now become the standard classification of sugars (Department of Health 1989).

> ### DISCUSSION POINTS
>
> List all the different terms that have been used to classify and name sugars. Identify the possible confusions created by the different names used.

The COMA classification is based upon where the sugar molecules are located within the food or drink structure (Fig. 12.1). Intrinsic sugars are found inside the cell structure of certain unprocessed foodstuffs, the most important being whole fruits and vegetables (containing mainly fructose, glucose, and sucrose). Extrinsic sugars, by contrast, are located outside the molecules of the foods and drinks. There are two types: milk extrinsic sugars and non-milk extrinsic sugars (NMES). The extrinsic milk sugars include lactose, found in dairy products such as milk and milk products. NMES are found in table sugar, confectionery, soft drinks, biscuits, honey, and fruit juice.

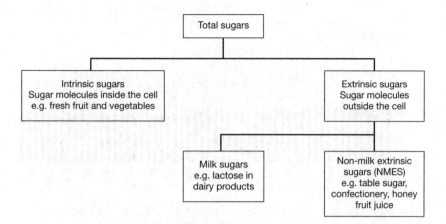

Fig. 12.1 Classification of sugar. (Reproduced from Watt 1999 with permission © HMSO. See Permissions.)

NMES CONSUMPTION PATTERNS WITHIN THE POPULATION

In the last 50 years patterns of eating have changed radically in the developed world. The types of foods and drinks consumed and the ways in which food is eaten have all changed. This has been caused by a wide range of social, economic, and political changes in society. The pattern of sugars consumption has been altered by these macro factors. Following the cessation of war-time rationing there was a massive increase in the consumption of sugars in the 1950s (Fig. 12.2). Since this peak in total consumption in the 1950s/1960s there has been a gradual reduction in the amount of NMES consumed. However, the pattern of consumption of NMES has changed greatly in the last 30 years. There has been a large reduction in consumption of table sugar (added to tea/coffee, breakfast cereals, etc.), and instead an increase in NMES contained in processed and manufactured foods and drinks (Sustain 2000).

Table 12.1 lists the NMES content of a range of popular foods and drinks.

The food industry spends large amounts of money each year on the promotion and advertising of sweetened products (Nielsen 1998). Fig. 12.3 provides details of advertising budgets on sugary foods and drinks.

EVIDENCE ON SUGARS AND CARIES

The relationship between sugars consumption and caries has been researched extensively for many years, and although the totality of the evidence is clear, the topic remains a keenly debated subject amongst certain interest groups.

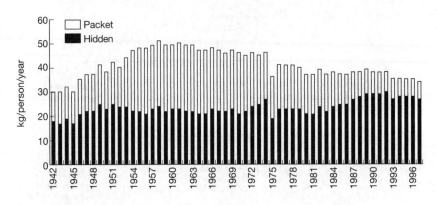

Fig. 12.2 Changing patterns of sugar consumption in the UK, 1942-96. (Reproduced with permission from Sustain 2000. See Permissions.)

DISCUSSION POINTS

In public health it is important to understand the range of perspectives on any given subject.
In connection to the relationship between sugar and caries, outline the range of groups who are most likely to have a keen interest in this subject.
Describe the key motivating factors behind these various interest groups.

The research evidence showing the relationship between sugars consumption and caries is based upon a range of different types of investigation (Box 12.1). (A very comprehensive and balanced review of the evidence is presented in Rugg-Gunn 1993.)

Table 12.1 NMES content of popular foods and drinks

Food/drink item	Percent NMES	Grams per serving
Coca Cola regular	10.5	35.0
Ribena regular	14.0	40.0
Lucozade regular	17.9	61.8
Sunny Delight	9.8	49.0
Nestlé Kit Kat	60.2	29.3
Fruit Pastilles	82.9	46.1
Kellogg's Frosties	38.0	11.2
Quaker Sugar Puffs	49.0	14.7
McVitie's Jaffa Cakes	52.0	13.0

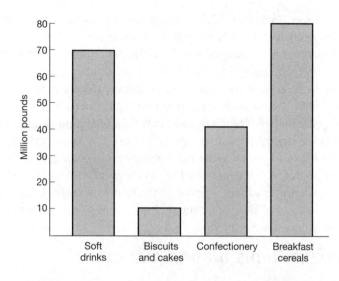

Fig. 12.3 Advertising budgets on sugars. (Reproduced with permission from Sustain 2000. See Permissions.)

DISCUSSION POINTS

What type of investigation would provide the best possible source of evidence to establish the relationship between sugars consumption and caries development?
Describe the design of such an investigation.
What are the problems with conducting such an investigation?

Box 12.1 Consensus view on diet and caries

- The influence of the diet is more important after the teeth have erupted. The pre-eruptive effect of diet on caries development is minimal.
- NMES are highly cariogenic.
- Frequency of eating/drinking NMES is important in caries development. However, frequency of intake and amount consumed are closely correlated.
- Intrinsic sugars, as found in, for example, fresh fruits and vegetables, and cooked staple starchy foods such as rice and potatoes, are of low cariogenicity. Milk extrinsic sugars, for example milk, are virtually non-cariogenic.
- Alternative or non-sugar sweeteners (bulk and intense) are non-cariogenic.

(Rugg-Gunn 1993.)

As can be seen from Box 12.2, a great deal of research has been conducted into assessing the relationship between caries and dietary factors. The different types of investigation have particular strengths and weaknesses. In isolation, evidence from only one type of investigation would be insufficient to determine the causation of caries. However, the combined results highlight a consensus view (Cannon 1992; Department of Health 1989; Rugg-Gunn 1993; Sheiham 2001; WHO 1990) and can be summarized as follows: sugars, particularly sucrose, are the most important dietary aetiological cause of caries. Both the frequency of consumption and total amount of sugars is important in the aetiology of caries. 'The evidence establishing sugars as an aetiological factor in dental caries is overwhelming. The foundation of this lies in the multiplicity of studies rather than the power of any one.' (Arens 1998)

RECOMMENDATIONS ON DIET AND CARIES

Based upon the available evidence the following consensus recommendations have been proposed (Department of Health 1989; WHO 1990):

- The frequency and amount of NMES should be reduced. NMES consumption should be restricted to mealtimes when possible.
- NMES should provide no more than 10% of total energy in the diet.
- Consumption of intrinsic sugars and starchy foods should be increased (5 pieces/portions of fruit/vegetable per day).

It is important to recognize that although plaque has an important role to play in the caries process there is insufficient evidence that plaque removal alone will reduce caries (Sutcliffe 1996). Tooth-brushing and professional cleaning are not capable of removing all the cariogenic microorganisms from the dentition. Tooth-brushing alone will not prevent caries. Using a fluoride toothpaste will, however, have a significant impact on the caries process.

DIETARY COUNSELLING IN THE DENTAL PRACTICE

As outlined in Chapter 10, helping patients to change their behaviour is not a simple task. In addition, from a public health perspective it is acknowledged that individualized health education will never tackle the underlying causes of disease in society and is often therefore largely ineffective (Sprod et al. 1996). However, dentists and their teams have a responsibility to help and support those of their patients who want and need to change their eating patterns. Effective dietary counselling should be developed from evidence-based guidelines as outlined in Box 12.1 and 12.3 (Roe et al. 1997).

Due to the demands on dentists' time and the fact that their expertise lies within clinical practice, dietary counselling is more often a responsibility of

Box 12.2 Different types of investigation and studies assessing the relationship between sugars and caries development

Observational human studies

World-wide epidemiology (Sreebny 1982).

Native populations, for example Inuit (Zitzow 1979).

Tristan da Cunha (Fisher 1968).

Groups eating low amounts of sugar.

    Hopewood House (Harris 1963).

    Hereditary fructose intolerance (Newbrun 1989).

    Dentists' children (Bradford and Crabb 1961).

    War-time diets (Takahashi 1961).

Groups eating high amounts of sugar

    Sugar-cane chewers (Frencken 1989).

    Workers in confectionery factories (Anaise 1978).

    Children taking sugar-based medicines (Roberts and Roberts 1979).

Interventional human studies

Vipeholm study (Gustaffson *et al.* 1954).

Turku study (Scheinin and Makinen 1975).

Recife study (Rogriques *et al.* 1999).

Animal experiments

Frequency of feeding (Konig *et al.* 1968).

Concentration of sugar (Shaw 1979).

Types of sugar (Grenby *et al.* 1973).

Enamel slab experiments

Lesion formation (Koulourides *et al.* 1976).

Plaque pH experiments

Acidogenicity tests (Imfeld 1977).

Incubation experiments

Test-tube experiments (Grenby *et al.* 1989).

(Rugg-Gunn 1993)

Box 12.3 Evidence-based dietary guidelines

• Interventions should be developed from behavioural theory and should incorporate well-defined goals. Information alone has only a limited impact.

• Personal contact is important in motivating and monitoring change. A detailed history is required to ascertain all relevant background information.

• Interventions should be tailored to individuals' personal circumstances and ability to change.

• Provision of feedback on dietary changes is important.

• Multiple contacts over a period of time are more likely to achieve desired goals.

• Encouragement and support from family and friends is essential to motivate and maintain change.

(Roe et al. *1997)*

other members of the dental team such as dental nurses, hygienists, and oral health promoters. It is essential, however, that the whole dental team participates. Dentists can take the lead in highlighting the need for dietary control through their clinical diagnosis. The more detailed and time consuming elements of counselling can then be taken over by the other team members.

DISCUSSION POINTS

Effective dietary counselling depends partly upon securing a detailed and appropriate diet history.
What types of information should be collected in a dietary history?
Design a method of collecting this information from a patient.
What are the main limitations of your suggested method?

Dietary advice given in the dental surgery will obviously be directed largely at preventing and controlling caries. It is vital, however, that all information given out is consistent with general health education messages. In the past the dental profession has been guilty of confusing the public by providing conflicting messages, the most obvious example being in relation to fat in the diet. Alternatives to sugary snacks and drinks should also not contain excessive levels of fat. Box 12.4 lists a collection of some recommended foods and drinks.

Box 12.4 Recommended foods and drinks

- Water
- Milk
- Diluted fruit juice
- Fresh fruit and vegetables
- Low fat unprocessed savoury foods
- Plain yogurt

COMMUNITY-WIDE INITIATIVES

Unhealthy eating practices will only ever be successfully changed through public health action (Love and Kalkins 1984). Based upon the principles of health promotion, population interventions to promote healthier eating should:

- **Focus:** address the underlying influences on food consumption and be aware of the barriers that prevent certain groups from adopting recommended diets.

Table 12.2 Food policy matrix

	Partners							
Intervention	Producers	Processors	Distributors	Catering	Consumers	Government	Media	Health services	Education and Social Services
Education								
Substitution								
Pricing								
Organizational policy								
Regulation								
Community action								

From Stockley 1993.

- **Evidence:** be evidence-based and ensure that recommendations are consistent and scientifically based.
- **Food chain**: adopt a multidisciplinary approach in which a range of relevant organizations, agencies, and professionals work together to promote healthier eating.
- **Action**: utilize a complementary range of health promotion strategies which move beyond a health education approach.

> ## DISCUSSION POINTS
>
> Many people have changed their eating habits in line with health advice. However, this is not universal.
> What groups in society tend to eat a less healthy diet?
> List the barriers that may prevent these groups from changing their eating habits.

Table 12.2 presents the range of strategies and partners that can be involved in a comprehensive public health nutrition programme.

CONCLUSION

Caries remains a significant public health problem, with the frequent consumption of NMES being the principal aetiological factor in its development. Dental professionals have a responsibility to assist their patients adopt healthier eating practices to maintain good oral health. Effective action can be delivered at both a clinical level and on a community basis.

REFERENCES

Anaise, J. (1978). Prevalence of dental caries among workers in the sweets industry in Israel. *Community Dentistry and Oral Epidemiology*, **6**, 286–89.

Arens, U. (1998). *Oral health, diet and other factors*. Amsterdam, Elsevier

Bradford, E. and Crabb, H. (1961). Carbohydrate restriction and caries incidence: a pilot study. *British Dental Journal*, **111**, 273–9.

Cannon, G. (1992). *Food and health: the experts agree*. London, Consumers Association.

Department of Health (1989). *Dietary sugars and human disease*. Committee on Medical Aspects of Food Policy. London, HMSO.

Fisher, F. (1968). A field study of dental caries, periodontal disease and enamel defects in Tristan da Cunha. *British Dental Journal*, **125**, 447–53.

Frencken, J., Rugarabamu, P. and Mulder, J. (1989). The effects of sugar cane chewing on the development of dental caries. *Journal of Dental Research*, **68**, 1102–4.

Grenby, T., Paterson, F. and Cawson, R. (1973). Dental caries and plaque formation from diets containing sucrose and glucose in gnotobiotic rats infected with Strepococcus strain IB-1600. *British Journal of Nutrition*, **29**, 221–8.

Grenby, T. Phillips, A. and Saldanha, M. (1989). The possible dental effect of children's rusks; laboratory evaluation by two different methods. *British Dental Journal*, **166**, 157–62.

Gustafsson, B., Quensel, C., Lanke, L. *et al*. (1954). The Vipeholm dental caries study. The effect of different levels of carbohydrate intake on caries activity in 436 individuals observed over five years. *Acta Odontology Scandinavia*, **11**, 232–364.

Harris, R. (1963). Biology of the children of Hopewood House, Bowral, Australia, 4. Observations on dental caries experience extending over five years (1957–1961). *Journal of Dental Research* **42**, 1387–99.

Imfeld, T. (1977). Evaluation of cariogenicity of confectionary by intraoral wire telemetry. *Helv Odontology Acta*, **21**, 1–28.

Konig, K. Schmid, P. and Schmid, R. (1968). An apparatus for frequency-controlled feeding of small rodents and its use in dental caries experiments. *Archives of Oral Biology*, **13**, 13–26.

Koulourides, T., Bodden, R., Keller, S. *et al*. (1976). Cariogenicity of nine sugars tested with an intraoral device in man. *Caries Research*, **10**, 427–41.

Love, R. and Kalkins, I. (1984). Individualist and structuralist perspectives on nutrition education for Canadian children. *Social Science and Medicine*, **18**, 199–204.

McDonald, S. and Sheiham, A. (1992). The distribution of caries on different tooth surfaces at varying levels of caries: a compilation of data from 18 previous studies. *Community Dental Health*, **9**, 39–48.

Mejare, I., Kallestal, C., Stenlund, H., and Johansson, H. (1998). Caries development from 11 to 22 years of age: a prospective radiographic study. *Caries Research*, **32**, 10–16.

Newbrun, E. (1989). *Cariology* (3rd Edn), Chicago, Quintessence.

Nielsen, C. (1998). *Marketing*, June 1998.

Roberts, I. and Roberts, G. (1979). Relation between medicines sweetened with sucrose and dental disease. *British Medical Journal*, **ii**, 14–16.

Rodrigues, C., Watt, R. G. and Sheiham, A. (1999). The effects of dietary guidelines on sugar intake and dental caries in 3 year olds attending nurseries. *Health Promotion International* **14**, 329–35.

Roe, L., Hunt, P., Bradshaw, H., and Rayner, M. (1997). *Health promotion interventions to promote healthy eating in the general population*. London, Health Education Authority.

Scheinin, A. and Makinen, K. (1975). Turku sugar studies. I–XXI. *Acta Odontology Scandinavia* **33**, Suppl, 1–349.

Shaw, J. (1979). Changing food habits and our need for evaluation of the cariogenic potential of foods and confections. *Pediatric Dentistry*, **1**, 192–8.

Sheiham, A. (2001). Dietary effects on dental diseases. *Public Health Nutrition*, **4**, 569–91.

Sprod, A., Anderson, R., and Treasure, E. (1996). *Effective oral health promotion*. [*Literature review*.] Cardiff, Health Promotion Wales.

Sreebny, L. (1982). The sugar-caries axis. *International Dental Journal*, **32**, 1–12.

Stockley, L. (1993). *Summary of the promotion of healthier eating: a basis for action*. London, Health Education Authority.

Sustain (Sustain: the alliance for better food and farming) (2000). *Sweet and sour: the impact of sugar production and consumption on people and the environment*. London, Sustain (www.sustainweb.org).

Sutcliffe, P. (1996). Oral cleanliness and dental caries. In *The prevention of oral disease* (ed. J. Murray), pp. 68–77. Oxford, Oxford University Press.

Takahashi, K. (1961). Statistical study on caries incidence in the first molar in relation to the amount of sugar consumption. *Bulletin Tokyo Dental College*, **1**, 58–70.

Watt, R. (ed.) (1999). *Oral health promotion: a guide to effective working in pre-school settings*. London, Health Education Authority.

WHO (World Health Organization) (1990). *Diet, nutrition and prevention of chronic diseases*. Geneva, WHO.

Zitzow, R. (1979). The relationship of diet and dental caries in the Alaskan eskimo population. *Alaska Medicine*, **21**, 10–14.

FURTHER READING

Rugg-Gunn, A. (1993). *Nutrition and dental health*. Oxford, Oxford University Press.

Rugg-Gunn, A. and Nunn, J. (1999). *Nutrition, diet and oral health*. Oxford, Oxford University Press.

13 Fluoride and fissure sealants

CONTENTS

By the end of this chapter you should be able to:

- Describe briefly how the action of fluoride was discovered.
- Describe how fluoride works in the prevention of dental caries.
- List and describe the methods of fluoride delivery.
- Be able to describe the advantages and disadvantages of each mode of delivery.
- Have an overview of the arguments for and against the use of fluoride in caries prevention.
- Outline the public health importance of fissure sealants.

This chapter links with:
- Trends on oral health (Chapter 6).
- Evidence-based dentistry (Chapter 7).
- Principles of oral health promotion (Chapter 9).
- Sugars and caries prevention (Chapter 12).

INTRODUCTION

Fluoride has made an enormous contribution to declines in dental caries over the past 60 years (Murray and Naylor 1996). Fissure sealants are a proven preventive agent. This chapter provides a brief overview of the history of fluoride and presents a brief synopsis of the mode of action, method of delivery, safety, and controversies in use of fluoride. A public health perspective on fissure sealants will also be presented.

FLUORIDE

The discovery of the action of fluoride: a brief history

A detailed account of the history of fluoride can be found in Murray *et al.* (1991) and Murray and Naylor (1996) and is summarized in this section (see Box 13.1 for key dates). In 1901, Frederick McKay, a dentist in Colorado Springs, USA noticed that many of his patients, who had spent all their lives in the area, had a distinctive stain on their teeth known locally as 'Colorado stain'. McKay was puzzled and called in the assistance of a dental researcher G. V. Black. They found that other communities in the USA had the characteristic mottling. Their histological examination of affected teeth showed that the enamel was imperfectly calcified, but that decay in the mottled teeth was no higher than in normal teeth.

McKay suspected that something in the water supply was producing the brown stain, and more evidence came from Bauxite, a community formed to house workers of a subsidiary of ALCOA (Aluminium Company of America). A local dentist noticed that children in Bauxite had mottled teeth whereas children in nearby Benton did not. McKay investigated the problem but was unable to find a cause for the staining when the water supply was tested. In 1933, Mr H. V. Churchill, Chief chemist for ALCOA (anxious that aluminium would not be blamed for the mottling) analysed the water and found that the fluoride ion concentration in the water supply of the Bauxite community was abnormally high (13.7 ppm). He tested other communities affected by mottling which had been previously identified by McKay and found that they too had high levels of fluoride present in the water supplies.

In 1938, after extensive surveys of all communities affected by mottling in the US, Dr H. Trendley Dean (a public health service scientist) summarized the knowledge in relation to tooth mottling and the presence of fluoride in the water. He showed that below a level of 1 ppm fluoride ion concentration, mottling disappeared or was minimal. Further studies in America showed that at a fluoride ion concentration of 1 ppm there was a reduction in caries, with no associated mottling of the teeth. All these findings had occurred in naturally fluoridated water supplies.

In 1944, Dean and co-workers began to test the safety of artificially fluoridating the water at 1 ppm, and in 1945 the water supply of Grand Rapids Michigan, was artificially fluoridated at this level. The town of Muskegon, Michigan was used as a control (that is, not fluoridated) and the town of Aurora, Illinois, which was naturally fluoridated, was also included in the study for comparative purposes. After 6 years of the study, F. A. Arnold, a co-worker of Dean, reported that the decay experience of children in Grand

---

Box 13.1 Key dates in the discovery of the action of fluoride

1902 Frederick McKay identifies 'Colorado stain' on the teeth of local residents.

1909 McKay undertakes a study describing the prevalence of the stain in the local community.

1933 Mr H. V. Churchill identifies the presence of fluoride in the water supply of Bauxite.

1938 H. Trendley Dean establishes that at levels of 1 ppm in naturally fluoridated communities, caries levels are low and there is no or minimal mottling of the teeth.

1953 F. A. Arnold reports that after 6 years of artificially fluoridating the water in Grand Rapids, USA, caries are reduced by half compared to the control group.

(Murray and Naylor 1996)

Rapids had declined by almost half compared to Muskegon and had similar levels to those seen in Aurora.

Fluoridation has therefore come to be defined as: 'controlled adjustment of a fluoride compound to a public water supply in order to bring the fluoride ion concentration up to a level which effectively prevents caries' (Burt and Eklund 1999). This figure is usually around 0.8–1 ppm in temperate climates. In hotter areas where more water is drunk, the level may be adjusted downwards to 0.5 ppm.

How does fluoride act in caries prevention?

There are three theories:
1. That fluoride becomes incorporated into the hydroxyapatite crystal and renders it more resistant to acid attack.
2. That the presence of saliva promotes remineralization of the early carious lesion.
3. That fluoride interferes with the metabolic pathways of bacteria, thus reducing acid.

There have been discussions in the literature about the pre- and post-eruptive effects of fluoride. The pre-eruptive effect refers to the chemical incorporation of fluoride into the tooth. The post-eruptive effect refers to the remineralization of early caries lesions (Murray and Naylor 1996). The post-eruptive effect is now considered the most important mode of action (Murray and Naylor 1996).

A distinction is also made between fluoride that is ingested systemically (through water fluoridation, milk, or salt fluoridation) and that which is applied topically (as toothpaste or gels, for example). Such distinctions are not helpful since, as has been noted by Murray and Naylor (1996), all methods of fluoride delivery can have both systemic and topical effects.

Methods of fluoride delivery

These are summarized in Box 13.2. It is important to carefully document all sources of fluoride before deciding to prescribe fluoride supplements to children or adults.

Safety of fluoridation

There have been claims that fluoridation causes cancer, Down's syndrome, and is environmentally unsound. Numerous studies have investigated the safety of fluoridation and found no evidence to support claims of harmful effects. The most recent legal case in the UK was the Strathclyde case in 1983. It made legal history as one of the longest court cases in British history. The presiding judge, Lord Jauncey, found the evidence for the safety of fluoridation to be convincing. However, the case for fluoridation failed on a legal technicality. In essence, the law as it then stood, although it has since been amended, did not permit the fluoridation of public water supplies. People who do not want to drink fluori-

Box 13.2 Methods of fluoride delivery

Fluoridation
- Life-long residency produces the greatest cario-protective effect.
- 20–40% reductions in caries over a lifetime.
- Over 250 million drink fluoridated water world-wide.
- 15% of UK water supplies are fluoridated.
- Caries increases after fluoridation cessation.
- Advantages: safe, cost-effective, consistent, good population coverage, compliance not needed, low risk of over dose.
- Disadvantages: freedom of choice removed; requires complex infrastructure and initial capital outlay.

Fluoride tablets and drops
- 40–50% reduction in caries experience in both adults and children.
- NaF is the compound of choice.
- Care required in prescribing to minimize over-dosage and fluorosis.
- 0.5 mgF/day in children 3 years and up.
- Advantages: effective, freedom of choice.
- Disadvantages: compliance needed, consistency of delivery needed, risk of overdose.

Fluoride salt
- Effective.
- Caries protective effect as good as fluoridation.
- Dose of 250 ppm in adults and less in children.
- Advantages: effective, freedom of choice, consistent and regular.
- Disadvantages: conflict with general health messages regarding reduction in salt intake and the prevention of coronary heart disease.

Fluoride milk
- Well absorbed, although calcium diminishes topical effect.
- Advantages: safe, effective, regular, consistent, freedom of choice, risk of overdose small.
- Disadvantages: untested in community settings.

Fluoride in fruit juices
- Few studies exist to support use.

Topical fluoride
- Examples include aqueous solutions of sodium fluoride and stannous fluoride, and low pH solutions such as the acidulated phosphate fluoride system.
- 20–35% reduction in caries.
- Used usually in school-based mouth-rinsing programmes.
- Varnishes may be applied directly to teeth in high concentrations when required.
- Advantages: effective, useful in individuals at high risk for dental caries, freedom of choice.
- Disadvantages: need personnel, time consuming, access to services.

Fluoride toothpastes
- Simplest method of fluoride delivery.
- World-wide declines in caries experience attributed to toothpastes.
- Typical concentrations used: 1000–1100 mg of flouride per gram of toothpaste; a lesser dose used in children.
- Advantages: easy, effective, freedom of choice.
- Disadvantages: toothpaste and toothbrushes expensive, risk of over-dosage.

(From Murray and Naylor 1996. Additional material from Burt and Eklund 1997; Groeneveld et al. *1990; Newbrun 1992; Van Eck 1987.)*

DISCUSSION POINTS

What factors would you consider when asked to prescribe fluoride drops by a mother of two children attending your practice. The children are boys aged 2 and 7 years.

dated water would not be able to have it removed from their water supply, thus their freedom to choose would be removed.

In *Saving lives: our healthier nation* (Department of Health 1999), the UK government announced that it was commissioning a systematic review of the evidence relating to the safety and effectiveness of water fluoridation. Systematic reviews differ from other types of review in that they adhere to strict scientific design in order to make them more comprehensive, to minimize the chance of bias, and so to ensure their reliability. The review was commissioned from the University of York (NHS Centre for Reviews and Dissemination 2000), and found that:

1. Fluoride was associated with a reduction in levels of dental caries.
2. There was a dose–response between the amount of fluoride in the water and the levels of fluorosis.
3. No other harmful effects were found.
4. Fluoride was still associated with reductions in caries even in later years when fluoride toothpaste was commonly used.
5. There was limited evidence to support the view that fluoridation reduced social inequalities.

DISCUSSION POINTS

Imagine you are a public health dentist who has been asked to present the case in favour of the introduction of fluoridation in your local city. What arguments would you put forward?
Now imagine you are a parent who is very concerned about local democracy and environmental issues. What arguments would you put forward to oppose fluoridation? Look at the arguments for and against fluoridation. Think carefully about the quality of the evidence you are using to support both claims. Try thinking about the evidence using an evidence-based approach.

Summary

Fluoridation and other forms of fluoride remain some of the most effective caries-preventive public health measures available. Their use has been shown to be safe and cost effective. However, their introduction into local communities can unleash powerful emotions around issues such as freedom of choice and local democracy. These issues are not trivial in the minds of the community and need to be handled sensitively so that people are exposed to evidence that allows them make an informed choice.

FISSURE SEALANTS

Fissure sealants are materials designed to be placed on the pits and fissures of molar teeth to prevent the development of dental caries. Clinical trials have demonstrated their effectiveness as a caries preventive agent but their use is still limited within dental services. Fissure sealants have great potential as a preventive measure but their use within public health programmes has certain limitations.

Fissure sealants as a clinical preventive agent

Fissure sealants have been used for over 20 years, and evidence from clinical trials and community-based interventions have demonstrated that they are an effective preventive agent (Ismail and Gagnon 1995; Messer *et al.* 1997). Light-curing and auto-polymerizing materials have been shown to equally effective. Within clinical practice, evidence-based guidelines have been produced to assist practitioners in the use of this agent (British Society of Paediatric Dentistry 2000).

The decision to apply a fissure sealant should be made on clinical grounds after a thorough clinical examination, supported by radiographs when necessary, and by indications of risk from the patient's medical, social, and family history (Box 13.3).

Fissure sealants as a public health measure

With the vast majority of carious lesions in the population now occurring in pits and fissures, fissure sealants could potentially be used as an effective public health measure in a targeted population approach.

CONCLUSION

Fluoride and fissure sealants are both effective caries preventive agents. In particular fluoride in toothpaste has made a major contribution to improvements in caries levels around the world. It is essential that the appropriate combinations of fluoride methods are used to ensure minimal risk of fluorosis. Clinicians should follow evidence-based guidelines on fissure sealant use.

Box 13.3 Recommendations for use of fissure sealants in clinical practice

Patient selection
- Children with special needs.
- Children with caries in their primary dentition (dmfs > 2).

Tooth selection
- When the above indications are met, all susceptible sites in permanent teeth should be sealed.
- Sealing of teeth should be undertaken whenever necessary, based upon regular assessment of relevant risk factors

Clinical circumstances
- Where doubt exists over the caries status of a susceptible site, a bite-wing radiograph should be taken. If it is certain that the carious lesion is confined to the enamel surface, a sealant should be placed and monitored closely. If caries is found to extend to dentine, a sealant restoration should be placed.

Follow-up
- All sealed surfaces should be regularly monitored, and radiographs taken at appropriate intervals.
- Any defective sealants should be repaired providing the area is caries free.

(Reproduced with permission from British Society of Paediatric Dentistry 2000)

DISCUSSION POINTS

What are the difficulties of using fissure sealants in a public health programme?
Consider some of the following issues:
- Access of most appropriate groups – addressing inequalities.
- Practical problems – application and monitoring procedures.
- Professional agenda – working with colleagues in the GDS.
- Long-term follow-up.

REFERENCES

British Society of Paediatric Dentistry (2000). A policy document on fissure sealants in paediatric dentistry. *International Journal of Paediatric Dentistry*, **10**, 174–7.

Burt, B. A. and Eklund, S. (1997). Community-based strategies for preventing dental caries. In *Community Oral Health* (ed. C. Pine) pp. 112–25, Oxford, Weight.

Department of Health (1999). *Saving lives: our healthier nation.* London, The Stationery Office.

Groeneveld, A., Van Ecyk, A., and Backer Dirks, O. (1990). Fluoride in caries prevention: is the effect pre- or post-eruptive? Journal of Dental Research, **69** (special issue), 751–5.

Ismail, A. and Gagnon, P. (1995). A longitudinal evaluation of fissure sealants applied in dental practice. *Journal of Dental Research*, **74**, 1583–90.

Messer, L., Calache, H. and Morgan, M. (1997). The retention of pit and fissure sealants placed in primary school children by Dental Health Services, Victoria. *Australian Dental Journal*, **42**, 233–9.

Murray, J. J. and Naylor, M. N. (1996). Fluorides and dental caries. In *The prevention of oral disease*, 3rd edn (ed. J. J. Murray), pp. 32–67. Oxford, Oxford University Press.

Murray, J., Rugg-Gunn, A., and Jenkins, G. (1991). *Fluorides in caries prevention* (3rd edn). London, Wright, Butterworth Heinemann.

Newbrun, E. (1992). Current regulations and recommendations concerning water fluoridation, fluoride supplements, and topical fluoride agents. *Journal of Dental Research*, **71**, 1255–65.

NHS Centre for Reviews and Dissemination (2000). *A systematic review of public water fluoridation*. York, NHS Centre for Reviews and Dissemination (Report 18).

Van Eck, A. (1987). Pre- and post-eruptive effect of fluoridated drinking water on dental caries experience. Thesis, University of Utrecht (NIPG-TNO no 87021).

FURTHER READING

British Society of Paediatric Dentistry (2000). A policy document on fissure sealants in paediatric dentistry. *International Journal of Paediatric Dentistry*, **10**, 174–7.

Murray, J. J. and Naylor, M. N. (1996). Fluorides in dental caries. In *The prevention of oral disease*, 3rd edn (ed. J. J. Murray), pp. 32–67. Oxford, Oxford University Press.

Murray, J., Rugg-Gunn, A., and Jenkins, G. (1991). *Fluorides in caries prevention* (3rd edn). London, Wright, Butterworth Heinemann.

NHS Centre for Reviews and Dissemination (2000). *A systematic review of public water fluoridation*. York, NHS Centre for Reviews and Dissemination (Report 18).

14 Prevention of periodontal diseases

CONTENTS

By the end of this chapter you should be able to:

- Describe the key epidemiological features of periodontal diseases.
- Outline the main aetiological factors in periodontal disease.
- Critically assess preventive options for periodontal disease.
- Outline preventive and health promotion approaches appropriate for the prevention of periodontal diseases.

This chapter links with:

- Public health approaches to prevention (Chapter 4)
- Overview of epidemiology (Chapter 5).
- Trends in oral health (Chapter 6).
- Principles of oral health promotion (Chapter 9).
- Oral health education in dental practice settings (Chapter 11).

INTRODUCTION

During the last 20 years our understanding of periodontal disease has been dramatically changed. Findings from clinical and epidemiological research have challenged the traditional progressive disease model and questioned the extent of destructive periodontal diseases within the population (Burt 1994; Locker *et al.* 1998; Sheiham 1991). Although gaps in our knowledge still exist about the precise nature and full extent of the condition, it is critically important that preventive and public health approaches to periodontal disease are based upon current scientific understanding of the condition. The chapter will therefore present an overview of current clinical and epidemiological research findings on periodontal disease. This will be followed by a critical review of the various options for prevention of the condition, with particular emphasis on the public health strategies required.

OVERVIEW OF EPIDEMIOLOGY OF PERIODONTAL DISEASE

Before considering the options for the prevention of periodontal diseases it is important to highlight the main epidemiological features of the condition.

A recent critical review of the epidemiological literature on periodontal disease drew the following conclusion:

> While moderate levels of attachment loss are to be found in a high percentage of middle aged and elderly subjects, severe loss is confined to a minority, albeit a substantial one. Severe loss is evident in only a few sites and, in general, affects only a small proportion of sites examined. (Locker *et al.* 1998)

Previously it was stated that periodontal disease is the major cause of tooth loss after the age of 40, but epidemiological evidence now clearly demonstrates that this is not the case (Burt 1994; Pilot 1997; Locker *et al.* 1998). Gingivitis may be widespread but in most cases this does not lead to premature tooth loss. Severe periodontal disease occurs in a few teeth in approximately 8–15% of the population in any given age cohort; the proportion affected, however, increases with age.

DISEASE PROCESS

During the 1960s and 197's periodontitis was considered to be a slowly and continually progressive condition. This *continuous progressive model* was based on the belief that gingivitis, once developed, would progress into the periodontium, leading to loss of attachment, bone destruction, and eventually loss of teeth. This was thought to affect all the teeth in the majority of the population and to be the main cause of tooth loss in adults. These conclusions, based on research using invalid measures of periodontal disease and on the erroneous interpretation of data from cross-sectional studies (Burt 1994), have now been largely dismissed.

The current concept of periodontal disease presents a very different model. Evidence now indicates that the disease has an episodic nature, in which short bursts of tissue destruction take place in certain teeth, in certain sites: the so-called *burst theories* (Goodson *et al.* 1982; Socransky *et al.* 1984). These short periods of disease activity are followed by longer periods of remission and healing. Although there is still much debate about models of progression, there is widespread consensus that loss of attachment is neither evenly distributed within the mouth nor the wider population (Pilot 1997). For the majority of the population progression of periodontal disease is very slow. An average rate of attachment loss of 0.05–0.10 mm per year has been demonstrated (Albander 1990; Selikowitz *et al.* 1981). Such a slow rate of progression means that most people will die before they have lost all their supporting alveolar bone.

AETIOLOGY

Although many factors are associated with periodontal disease, dental plaque is considered to be its most important cause (Box 14.1). The more

---

Box 14.1 Primary causes of periodontal disease

- Plaque
- Smoking
- Systemic infections, for example, diabetes, HIV
- Stress
- Genetic disorders
- Factors predisposing to plaque accumulation:
    Overhanging restorations
    Removable partial dentures
    Calculus
    Tooth malalignment

---

plaque on the teeth, the greater the amount of disease present. The plaque–periodontal disease relationship is S-shaped. There is a level of plaque which does not lead to significant disease progression. The gingivitis related to this low level has been termed 'contained gingivitis'. Beyond this level, the more plaque in the mouth, the more disease. This linear, straight-line relationship exists to a certain point, beyond which an increase in plaque no longer affects disease levels (Sheiham 1991). In addition to the amount of plaque present, the nature and efficacy of local and systemic host responses to the pathogenic microbes in plaque is also an important and complex factor in determining disease progression.

From a public health perspective the other important aetiological factor associated with destructive periodontal disease is smoking. Tobacco smoking, in addition to being a key aetiological factor for oral cancer, is now associated with aggravated periodontal breakdown (Legarth and Reibel 1998). Smoking should therefore be seen as an important focus for preventive action by the dental team.

Other factors associated with increased susceptibility to destructive periodontal disease include certain systemic diseases, for example, diabetes and HIV infection, stressful life events, genetic disorders, and local factors predisposing to plaque accumulation. The presence of calculus (calcified plaque) has often been considered as a direct cause of periodontal disease, but there is no evidence that calculus itself is capable of initiating it (Jenkins 1996). Calculus is an inert substance; the surface texture of calculus, however, promotes plaque retention and accumulation.

IMPACT ON INDIVIDUAL AND SOCIETY

As outlined in Chapter 1, to decide if a condition can be regarded as a public health problem the impact of the disease on both the individual and society needs to be considered.

PREVENTIVE STRATEGIES

Goals for prevention

In any preventive strategy it is critical that clear and realistic targets are set. This is important in determining the selection of appropriate actions and devising relevant evaluation systems. In the prevention of periodontal disease it is vital to have targets that are based on up-to-date knowledge of the disease process and contemporary epidemiological data. If the overall aim of a dental public health strategy is the maintenance of a functional, and aesthetically and socially acceptable, natural dentition for the lifespan of most people, how can this be translated into a suitable goal for periodontal health?

Wennstrom *et al.* (1990) have proposed the following:

> The control of the development of destructive disease in order to prevent loss of function of the tooth/dentition throughout life, rather than the prevention and/or elimination of all clinical signs of periodontal inflammation.

This acknowledges that a plaque-free mouth is neither realistic nor necessary. Instead, some plaque, calculus, gingivitis, and attachment loss can be considered acceptable as long as this does not endanger the survival of the dentition. Based upon this principle a decision-making model for periodontal care has been proposed (Wennstrom *et al.* 1990). This states that a suitable goal for periodontal health would be alveolar bone height at the age of 75 years corresponding to at least one-third of the root length, based upon an estimated bone height at 25 years of age.

WHO (1982) have proposed a set of age-related goals for periodontal health, which are outlined in Table 14.1.

Table 14.1 Acceptable levels of periodontal status

Age (years)	Periodontal status
12	0 teeth with pockets > 3 mm
15	0 teeth with pockets > 3 mm
18	0 teeth with pockets > 3 mm
35–44	< 7 teeth with pockets > 4.5 mm
65–74	20 functional teeth

From WHO 1982.

Strategy selection

As outlined in Chapter 4, the medical and dental professions traditionally have tended to concentrate on a high-risk preventive strategy (Rose 1985). The limitations of this are now well recognized and the example of periodontal disease prevention provides a good example of the problems with adopting only a high-risk approach.

The success of the high-risk approach depends upon being able to identify individuals at particular risk of developing future disease at an early stage when intervention will alter the natural history of the condition (Rose 1985). A screening test with a high sensitivity and specificity is therefore essential. Although there is currently a great deal of research into periodontal disease predictors, at present no screening test is available that can be recommended for use in clinical settings or in population screening programmes (Pilot 1997). At present the best predictor of future breakdown is past experience of disease.

The limitations of the high-risk approach highlight the need to focus on a population strategy. Such an approach, by addressing the underlying causes of the problem (in this case plaque levels and smoking), reduces the risk for the whole population and therefore produces a greater benefit overall (Rose 1985). A modified approach, the targeted-population strategy, can also be used to direct action at particular high-risk groups within the population (but not individuals). The following two sections will outline possible preventive measures at both a clinical and population level.

Health education in clinical practice

Dentists and their team members have a professional responsibility to impart to their clients the knowledge and skills required to perform effective oral hygiene self-care practices. This is the only rational long-term method of controlling plaque. As was outlined in Chapter 10, a change in behaviour,

---

Box 14.2 Key health education messages to promote periodontal health

- Children under 7 years should be supervised with their brushing.
- Gentle scrub technique is an effective tooth-brushing method.
- Gentle pressure – hold brush with a pen grip.
- Use of floss, sticks, and interdental aides are optional and need professional advice.
- Toothbrush size: use a small head with soft to medium texture.
- Replace toothbrush when bristles become excessively splayed.
- Chlorhexidine is the most effective chemical plaque suppressant.

(Levine 1996)

---

such as a modified tooth-brushing technique, requires more than just a leaflet with some information. Effective tooth-cleaning is a skill which requires detailed instruction, practice, and feedback (see Box 14.2).

Health education directed at improving oral hygiene should be provided in a supportive and personalized format which recognizes the individual's concerns and circumstances. The public may have good rational reasons for not complying with professional recommendations (Nettleton 1986). Effective communication skills are an essential requirement in this process; as well as verbal advice, high-quality health education materials such as leaflets can also be an important source of additional help and support.

DISCUSSION POINTS

Outline the different steps involved in giving oral hygiene instruction (OHI)? What ways would you suggest to evaluate the effectiveness of clinical OHI?

For the small number of people with rapidly destructive disease, more intensive therapy and support will be required. Appropriate anti-microbial therapy and surgical treatment can then also be offered. However, this intensive dentist-based approach is not required for the majority of the population, being both very expensive and time consuming (Sheiham 1991).

Public health approaches

The most significant means of preventing periodontal disease will be achieved through population-based methods aimed at reducing overall plaque levels and smoking rates (see Box 14.3).

Mouth feel, freshness, mouth smell, and appearance are the common reasons for tooth-brushing (Gift 1986). Mouth-cleaning is part of personal hygiene and grooming behaviour, and therefore has a strong social motivation rather than purely a health focus (Hodge *et al.* 1982). Isolated one-off

---

Box 14.3 Public health measures to reduce periodontal diseases

- Integrate oral hygiene into body cleanliness education at nurseries and schools.
- Incorporate the importance and skills of oral hygiene into training of health, education, and social care professionals.
- Use fiscal policy to reduce costs of oral hygiene aids and toothpaste: remove VAT at national level and/or sell products at cost price within NHS premises.
- Organizational policy: ensure oral hygiene is placed on health-promoting schools' agendas – structural change within schools regarding provision and design of toilet facilities.
- Comprehensive public health strategies to reduce smoking, especially amongst low income groups.

---

campaigns specifically designed to improve oral hygiene do not produce long-term sustainable changes in behaviour and are very costly (Kay and Locker 1996; Sprod *et al.* 1996). Instead, schemes to promote oral cleanliness should be incorporated into health education programmes that are aiming to improve body cleanliness and grooming. This integrated approach, based upon sound educational theory, is far more likely to produce long-term behaviour modification, partly through the impact of primary and secondary socialization on behaviour. In addition, professional education on tooth-cleaning practices to influential professional groups such as health visitors, pharmacists, and teachers may be a far more effective means of disseminating a message to the general public than direct contact.

Environmental and structural factors also have an important role to play in promoting periodontal health. For example, the provision of appropriate hygiene facilities within schools, factories, and offices may encourage tooth-cleaning. Many oral hygiene aides are currently very expensive, and for a family on a low income a new toothbrush is unlikely to be a major priority. Marketing practices which promote high-quality, low-cost oral hygiene products could be particularly important in areas of deprivation.

Potentially, the most significant development to affect population plaque levels is not related to any health promotion intervention per se, but due instead to the commercial marketing and sales of newly developed anti-plaque and anti-calculus toothpastes by toothpaste manufacturers. Rather like the decline in caries, plaque levels may be significantly reduced by changes in commercial product formulation rather than dentists' efforts.

CONCLUSION

The epidemiological data on periodontal disease highlights that the severe destructive form is relatively rare, and that the condition is not the most important cause of tooth loss for the majority of adults. Dental plaque and smoking are the two most significant aetiological factors. Traditional clinical approaches to the prevention of periodontal disease are very expensive and most unlikely to successfully treat the condition at a population level. Public health approaches to plaque and smoking reduction offer far greater benefits at reduced cost.

REFERENCES

Albander, J. (1990). A 6 year study on the pattern of periodontal disease progression. *Journal of Clinical Periodontology*, **17**, 467–71.

Burt, B. (1994). Periodontitis and aging: reviewing recent evidence. *Journal of American Dental Association*, **125**, 273–9.

Gift, H. (1986). Current utilization patterns of oral hygiene practices. In *Dental plaque control measures and oral hygiene practices* (ed. H. Loe and D. Kleinman), pp. 31–71. Oxford, IRL Press.

Goodson, J., Tanner, A., Haffajee, A., *et al.* (1982). Patterns of progression and regression of advanced destructive periodontal disease. *Journal of Clinical Periodontology*, **9**, 472–81.

Hodge, H., Holloway, P., and Bell, C. (1982). Factors associated with tooth brushing behaviours in adolescents. *British Dental Journal*, **152**, 49–51.

Jenkins, W. (1996). The prevention and control of chronic periodontal disease. In *Prevention of oral disease* (ed. J. Murray), pp. 118–38. Oxford, Oxford University Press.

Kay, L. and Locker, D. (1996). Is dental health education effective? A systematic review of current evidence. *Community Dentistry and Oral Epidemiology*, **24**, 231–5.

Legarth, J. and Reibel, J. (1998). EU Working Group on Tobacco and Oral Health. *Oral Diseases*, **4**, 48–67.

Levine, R. (1996). *The scientific basis of dental health education: a policy document* (4th edn). London, Health Education Authority.

Locker, D., Slade, G., and Murray, H. (1998). Epidemiology of periodontal disease among older adults: a review. *Periodontology 2000*, **16**, 16–33.

Nettleton, S. (1986). Understanding dental health beliefs: an introduction to ethnography. *British Dental Journal*, **161**, 145–7.

Pilot, T. (1997). Public health aspects of oral disease and disorders: periodontal diseases. In *Community oral health* (ed. C. M. Pine), pp. 82–8. London, Wright.

Rose, G. (1985). Sick individuals and sick populations. *International Journal of Epidemiology*, **14**, 32–8.

Selikowitz, H., Sheiham, A., Albert, D., and Williams, G. (1981). Retrospective longitudinal study of the rate of alveolar bone loss in humans using bite-wing radiographs. *Journal of Clinical Periodontology*, **8**, 431–8.

Sheiham, A. (1991). Public health aspects of periodontal diseases in Europe. *Journal of Clinical Periodontology*, **18**, 362–9.

Socransky, S., Haffajee, A., Goodson, J., and Linde, J. (1984). New concepts of destructive periodontal disease. *Journal of Clinical Periodontology*, **11**, 21–32.

Sprod, A., Anderson, R., and Treasure, E. (1996). *Effective oral health promotion.* [Literature review.] Cardiff, Health Promotion Wales.

Wennstrom, J., Papapanou, P., and Grondahl, K. (1990). A model for decision making regarding periodontal treatment needs. *Journal of Clinical Periodontology*, **17**, 217–22.

WHO (World Health Organization) (1982). *A review of current recommendations for the organization and administration of community oral health services in Northern and Western Europe. Report of a WHO Workshop.* Copenhagen, WHO Regional Office for Europe.

FURTHER READING

Jenkins, W. (1996). The prevention and control of chronic periodontal disease. In *Prevention of oral disease* (ed. J. Murray), pp. 118–38. Oxford, Oxford University Press.

Locker, D., Slade, G., and Murray, H. (1998). Epidemiology of periodontal disease among older adults: a review. *Periodontology 2000*, **16**, 16–33.

Pilot, T. (1997). Public health aspects of oral disease and disorders: periodontal diseases. In *Community oral health* (ed. C. M. Pine), pp. 82–8. Oxford, Wright.

15 Oral cancer prevention

CONTENTS

By the end of this chapter you should be able to:

- Outline the principal epidemiological facts for oral cancer in the UK.
- Describe the aetiology of oral cancer.
- Identify opportunities for prevention of oral cancer within the clinical environment.
- Outline a range of public health approaches to oral cancer prevention.

This chapter links with:
- Introduction to the principles of public health (Chapter 1).
- Determinants and definitions of oral health (Chapters 2 and 3).
- Public health approaches to prevention (Chapter 4).
- Principles of oral health promotion (Chapter 9).
- Overview of behaviour change (Chapter 10).
- Oral health education in dental practice settings (Chapter 11).

INTRODUCTION

Oral cancer is one of the few conditions that dental professionals may encounter within their surgeries which can be fatal. It is therefore essential that members of the dental team understand the epidemiology and natural history of the condition and possible options for prevention, screening, and treatment.

From a public health perspective oral cancer presents many interesting challenges. Firstly, is the condition a public health problem? In this chapter the epidemiology of oral cancer will be reviewed to highlight the extent and impact of the condition. Secondly, what options exist to prevent the disease and how best can these be implemented? As we will discuss, although progress has been made in the treatment of the disease, survival rates have not improved substantially in recent decades (Cancer Research Campaign 2000; Stell and McCormick 1985). The potential for screening of the condition has been extensively reviewed, and currently a national screening programme is not recommended due to a lack of evidence on effectiveness (Chamberlain 1993). Although various initiatives have recently attempted to co-ordinate and expand the prevention of oral cancer (British Dental Association 1998), the preventive activities presently undertaken by the dental profession alone are unlikely to be successful. A clear need exists for a comprehensive public health strategy to tackle the underlying causes of the disease in a co-ordinated fashion. This chapter will therefore outline the scope and detail of such a strategy.

EPIDEMIOLOGY OF ORAL CANCER

Incidence

Oral cancers commonly include cancer of the lip, tongue, mouth, and pharynx. In the UK there are approximately 3500 new cases of, and 1600 deaths from oral cancer each year. The disease is almost twice as common in men as in women, and the majority of malignancies are squamous cell carcinomas. The incidence increases with age, and 85% of cases in the UK are found in people aged over 50 years (Cancer Research Campaign 2000). Regional variations exist across the country with a higher incidence in Scotland, Northern Ireland, and Wales compared to England. Significant socio-economic inequalities exist in oral cancer rates (Edwards and Jones 1999). As shown in Fig. 15.1, this association is especially strong for men, in which the risk of developing cancer of the oral cavity is over four times greater in the most deprived populations compared to more affluent groups (Harris *et al.* 1998).

Internationally the incidence varies considerably, with very high rates found particularly in India and Sri Lanka, where oral malignancy is the commonest type of cancer, accounting for 40% of all cancers. In the UK, oral cancers account for 1–2% of all new cases of cancer, similar to multiple myeloma and cervical cancer.

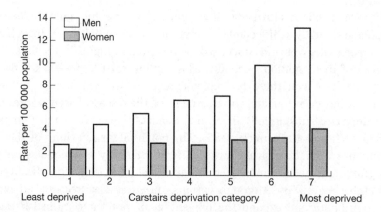

Fig. 15.1 Incidence rates of oral cancer by deprivation, 1986-95. (Reproduced from CRC CancerStat report, with permission from the Cancer Research Campaign 2000. See Permissions.)

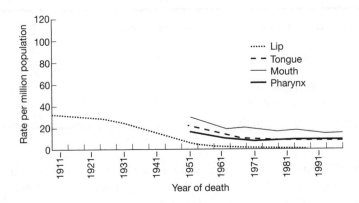

Fig. 15.2 Age-standardized mortality rates for male cancer of the lip, tongue, mouth and pharynx, England and Wales, 1911-98. (Reproduced from CRC CancerStat report, with permission from the Cancer Research Campaign 2000. See Permissions.)

Trends

As Fig. 15.2 shows, a striking decrease in mortality for male oral cancers took place between 1911 and the early 1970s. For example, the age-standardized mortality rates per million population for cancers of the tongue decreased from 67 to 6 (Cancer Research Campaign 2000).

DISCUSSION POINTS

What possible explanations could be proposed to explain the dramatic decline in oral cancer between 1911 and the early 1970s?
Address this question from a public health perspective and consider what evidence you have to back up your ideas.

In recent years, however, there are indications that the incidence and mortality rates have started to increase, especially amongst younger men (Boyle *et al.* 1993; Hindle *et al.* 1994; Macfarlane *et al.* 1992; Osmond *et al.* 1983). The reason for this change is not clear.

LIMITATIONS OF TREATMENT

Although advances in technology and surgical techniques may have improved the quality of life for people affected by oral cancer, no marked improvements in cure rates have been detected in recent decades (Stell and McCormick 1985). The 5-year survival rate is only 50%, although this improves to 80% when the lesion is detected at an early stage (British Dental Association 1998; Cancer Research Campaign 2000). Survival rates for cancers of the tongue, oropharynx, and oral cavity vary significantly

Box 15.1 Factors influencing survival from oral cancer

- Site of lesion (the further back in the mouth, the poorer the prognosis).
- Size of lesion.
- Degree of differentiation.
- Involvement of regional lymph nodes.
- Presence of distant metastases.

between different socio-economic groups, with the most disadvantaged patients dying sooner than more affluent ones (Coleman *et al.* 1999).

The ability to detect lesions at a very early stage is crucial for the effective treatment of the disease (Box 15.1).

AETIOLOGY

The cause of oral cancer is largely understood and many cases could be prevented if the appropriate measures were undertaken. The key aetiological factors associated with the development of oral cancer are listed in Box 15.2.

The two most important risk factors associated with oral cancer are high consumption of tobacco and alcohol, which together cause 75–90% of all cases. These factors act synergistically to multiply the risk of oral cancer, as shown in Fig. 15.3.

Tobacco can be used in several ways. In the UK cigarette smoking is the most common form of tobacco use, but the habit is not practised evenly across the population. Since the 1960s smoking has become increasingly associated with social deprivation and poverty. In 1996, 12% of men in pro-

Box 15.2 Aetiology of oral cancer

Established risk factors
- Smoking tobacco.
- Chewing tobacco/oral snuff.
- Chewing betel quid (pan) with tobacco.
- Heavy consumption of alcohol.
- Presence of potentially malignant lesions.

Predisposing factors
- Dietary deficiencies (vitamins A, C, and E, and iron).
- Genetic disposition.
- Sunlight (lip cancer).
- Dental trauma.
- Viral infections.

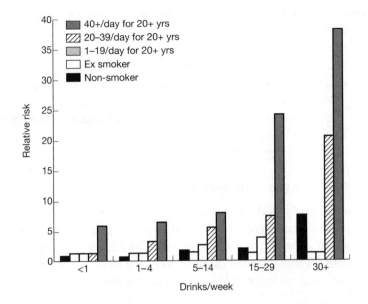

Fig. 15.3 Relative risk of oral/pharyngeal cancer in males by alcohol/tobacco consumption using US measures. (Reproduced from CRC CancerStat report, with permission from the Cancer Research Campaign 2000. See Permissions.)

fessional occupations smoked compared with 40% in unskilled manual jobs (Thomas *et al.* 1998). Increasingly, smoking is becoming restricted to more disadvantaged groups in society.

Tobacco can also be chewed alone or added to betel quid (pan). These habits have a strong cultural basis and are common amongst certain minority ethnic groups (Johnson and Warnakulasuriya 1993). Alcohol consumption in the UK doubled between the 1950s and the 1990s from 3.9 to 7.8 litres per head per year and there has been a steady shift in consumption away from beers to wines and spirits (Brewers Society 1999).

Diets low in vitamins A, C, and E have been associated with an increased risk of developing oral cancers (McLaughlin *et al.* 1988). Indeed, strong evidence exists to demonstrate that the antioxidants in fresh fruits and vegetables provide a protective function in the prevention of many types of cancers (Doll 1992). It is now recommended that at least five portions of fruit or vegetables should be consumed each day.

Certain oral lesions such as leukoplakia (white patches) and erythroplakia (red patches) can precede the development of malignancies. However, the rate of malignant transformation is very low, at 2–6%.

PREVENTIVE OPTIONS

The treatment of oral cancer is expensive for society, and for the individual affected the impact in terms of physical, psychological, and emotional costs is considerable; yet the prognosis is still poor. However, at least three-quarters of oral cancers could be prevented if tobacco and alcohol consumption were better controlled (Cancer Research Campaign 2000). The importance of developing and implementing effective and appropriate preventive measures is therefore obvious. The dental profession has tended to focus attention at an individual level and especially on the need for oral cancer screening. Although preventive action at a clinical level is important, there is also a need for a broader public health strategy which addresses the underlying cause of oral cancer.

To screen or not to screen, that is the question

A recent UK working group considered the possibility of recommending a national screening programme for oral cancer (Speight *et al.* 1993). The expert group concluded that due to insufficient evidence on the costs, benefits, effectiveness, feasibility, and appropriateness of screening for oral cancer, such a programme could not be recommended.

DISCUSSION POINTS

Outline the principles of screening?
How does the screening of oral cancer comply with these principles?
What further research is required before a national oral cancer screening programme could be recommended?

A CLINICAL APPROACH TO THE PREVENTION OF ORAL CANCER

Comprehensive medical history

A comprehensive and thorough medical history should always be taken with all new patients, and at recall-appointments for existing patients. All practitioners should routinely ask their patients about their tobacco and alcohol habits. This information should be recorded in the patient notes and referred to at subsequent appointments when appropriate.

Detailed and thorough oral examination

Although a national screening programme for oral cancer cannot be currently recommended, the value of opportunistic screening should be stressed (British Dental Association 1998). A thorough and detailed extra- and intra-oral examination of the hard and soft tissues should therefore be undertaken during dental check-ups, especially for those at greater risk of oral cancer. These include men aged 50 years and over, smokers and heavy drinkers, people who regularly chew betel quid (pan) with tobacco, patients with a history of cancer, and those with leukoplakia and erythroplakia.

Patient counselling

The dental team have an important role to play in advising and supporting their patients in adopting healthier choices. In the prevention of oral cancer three key messages need to be stressed:

1. Stop smoking.
2. Be moderate in alcohol use (3–4 units daily for men and 2–3 units daily for women).
3. It is important to eat five or more portions of fresh fruit and vegetables a day.

Smoking is an addictive behaviour with strong social associations and is very difficult to stop. However, advice, support, and encouragement from primary health care professionals can have a significant impact for those who want to quit. Although relatively few well-designed studies have assessed the effectiveness of smoking cessation initiated in dental practice settings, the available evidence suggests that success rates similar to other primary care settings can be achieved (Cohen *et al.* 1989; Smith *et al.* 1998). It has been estimated that between 63 000 and 190 000 smokers would stop smoking in a year if all dentists routinely offered smoking cessation advice (Watt *et al.* 2000).

DISCUSSION POINTS

Outline the range of reasons why people may start to smoke.
Most people are fully aware of the health risks of smoking, so what factors prevent individuals from successfully quitting?

Smoking cessation is one of the few areas of health promotion where good evidence exists to demonstrate effectiveness (Raw *et al.* 1998). It is therefore very important that members of the dental team become involved in smoking cessation activity within their practices. Simple, tailored questioning, advice, and follow-up support are all that is required to help patients successfully stop smoking. Figure 15.4 outlines the recommended protocol for effective smoking-cessation support based upon the '4As' model (Watt and Robinson 1999).

Another important opportunity for the dental team is in advising young people not to experiment with cigarettes. Most smokers start the habit when they are 11–14 years old, and once they are smoking a few cigarettes, many then become addicted to nicotine and find it very difficult to quit. The dental team are in a unique position to influence this age group as many young people will have little contact with other members of the health team. In addition, the immediate effects of smoking on the mouth, such as stained teeth and halitosis, may be a concern for many people and therefore a useful motivating factor to quit.

The Four As

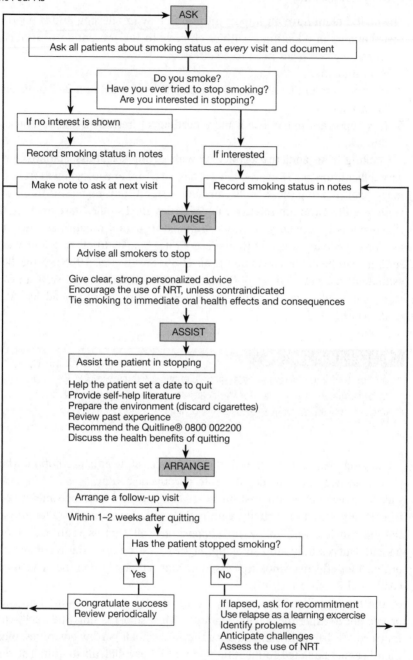

Fig. 15.4 Smoking cessation protocol. (Reproduced with permission from Watt and Robinson 1999 with permission © HMSO. See Permissions.)

Prompt and appropriate referral

It is essential that practitioners should request an urgent specialist appointment for any patient with a lesion which is suspected of malignancy. Prompt referral is critical as any delay may affect the long-term prognosis. Clear and concise details within the referral letter aid the referral process. Increasing numbers of specialist cessation-counselling centres have been established across the country to provide more intensive support for people unable to give up smoking.

PUBLIC HEALTH APPROACH

Due to the recognized limitations of current treatment modalities and the difficulty of introducing a comprehensive screening programme, the only means of significantly reducing the incidence of oral cancer is through the development of a public health strategy. The British government has recently published a comprehensive strategy aimed at reducing smoking rates across the population, and in particular amongst young people, pregnant women, and those living in deprived communities (Department of Health 1998).

In line with the principles of health promotion outlined in Chapter 9 a public health strategy to reduce oral cancer should be based upon the following principles:

- An understanding of the *underlying social, economic, and political determinants* of oral cancer; that is, the broad range of factors influencing tobacco and alcohol use and the barriers to increasing fruit and vegetable consumption.
- A *directed population approach* which targets action at high-risk groups and addresses health inequalities. (A high-risk approach is not applicable due to the limitations of current screening methods.)
- It should be based upon a *common risk-factor approach* in which dental health professionals collaborate with other health professionals to address common threats to oral and general health, for example, tobacco and alcohol.
- It recognizes the need to work in *partnerships* across sectors and agencies beyond health services.
- It should be based upon the need to work with *community members*, addressing their concerns and jointly tackling the underlying causes of the problem.
- It stresses the importance of utilizing a *range of complementary health promotion approaches* beyond a sole reliance on health education (see Box 15.3).

DISCUSSION POINTS

What sectors and agencies outside the health services could contribute to an oral cancer public health strategy?
What incentives could be used to encourage these groups to become involved in such a strategy?

Based upon the Ottawa Charter (WHO 1986), Box 15.3 outlines a range of options for a public health approach to oral cancer prevention.

Box 15.3 Public health approaches to oral cancer prevention

Build healthy public policy
- Tighten restrictions on tobacco and alcohol advertising and promotion.
- Fiscal policy: subsidize the costs of healthier choices, for example fruit and vegetables, and smoking substitutes (Nicotine Replacement Therapy).
- Improve labelling on betel quid products.

Create supportive environments
- Smoke-free public spaces, for example cinemas.
- Increase availability of fresh fruit and vegetables – school canteens and tuckshops.

Strengthen community action
- Promote establishment of local community-based smoking-cessation support groups.
- Establish help-lines which appeal to population groups with high rates of smoking.
- Support establishment of local food co-operatives selling cheap high-quality fruit and vegetables.

Develop personal skills
- Expand personal and social education in schools – life skills – empowerment, refusal and negotiation skills, etc.
- Incorporate tobacco and alcohol control within Health Promoting Schools initiatives.

Reorient health services
- Expand health professionals' education and training in smoking cessation and alcohol control.
- Increase numbers and range of health promotion professionals within the NHS with expertise in smoking and alcohol support.
- Establish evidence-based smoking and alcohol preventive services within primary care settings.

(Based on WHO 1986.)

DISCUSSION POINTS

An innovative health promotion programme in east London has attempted to work with the local community to reduce the oral health risks associated with betel quid (pan) chewing (Croucher and O'Farrell 1998).

Based upon the principles of health promotion, outline the approach you would recommend for an oral cancer strategy in community such as east London.

CONCLUSION

Although the number of oral cancer cases in the UK is relatively small, the impact of the disease on individuals affected and the wider society is great. Advances in treatments may have improved the quality of life of oral cancer suffers but survival rates have remained largely unchanged for several decades. A national screening programme is not currently recommended due to the limitations of available detection methods. The cause of the disease is, however, well established and the potential for effective prevention is considerable. A greater emphasis needs to be placed upon implementing evidence-based preventive measures within clinical dental settings. In addition, there is a need for a supporting public health strategy to address the wider social, economic, and political determinants of oral cancer.

REFERENCES

Boyle, P., Macfarlane, G., and Scully, C. (1993). Oral cancer: necessity for prevention strategies. *Lancet*, **342**, 1129.

British Dental Association (1998). *Oral Cancer: guidelines for early detection.* BDA Occasional Paper, Issue Number 5. London, British Dental Association.

Cancer Research Campaign (2000). *CRC CancerStats: Oral – UK.* London, Cancer Research Campaign.

Chamberlain, J. (1993). Evaluation of screening for cancer. *Community Dental Health*, **10** (Suppl. 1), 5–11.

Cohen, S., Stookey, G., Katz, B., *et al.* (1989). Helping smokers quit: a randomised controlled trial with private practice dentists. *Journal of American Dental Association*, **118**, 41–5.

Coleman, M., Babb, P., Damiecki, P., *et al.* (1999). *Cancer survival trends in England and Wales 1971–1995: deprivation and NHS region.* London, The Stationery Office.

Croucher, R. and O'Farrell, M. (1998). *Community based prevention of oral cancer: health promotion strategies relating to betel quid chewing in east London.* London, St Bartholomew's and the Royal London School of Medicine and Dentistry.

Department of Health (1998). *Smoking kills: a white paper on tobacco.* London, The Stationery Office.

Doll, R. (1992). The lessons of life: keynote address to the Nutrition and Cancer conference. *Cancer Research*, **52**, 2024–9.

Edwards, D. and Jones, J. (1999). Incidence of and survival from upper aerodigestive tract cancers in the UK: the influence of deprivation. *European Journal of Cancer*, **35**, 968–72.

Harris, V., Sandridge, A., Black, R., *et al.* (1998). *Cancer registration statistics Scotland 1986–1995*. Edinburgh, ISD Scotland Publications.

Hindle, I., Downer, M., and Speight, P. (1994) Necessity for prevention strategies in oral cancer. *Lancet*, **343**, 178–9.

Johnson, N. W. and Warnakulasuriya, K. A. A. S. (1993). Epidemiology and aetiology of oral cancer in the United Kingdom. *Community Dental Health*, **10** (Suppl. 1), 13–29.

Macfarlane, G., Boyle, P., and Scully, C. (1992). Oral cancer in Scotland: changing incidence and mortality. *British Medical Journal*, **305**, 1121–3.

McLaughlin, J. K., Gridley, G., Block, G., *et al.* (1988). Dietary factors in oral and pharyngeal cancer. *Journal of the National Cancer Institute*, **80**, 1237–43.

Osmond, C., Gardner, M., Acheson, E., and Adelstein, A. (1983) *Trends in cancer mortality, England and Wales 1951–1980*. HMSO Series DH1 No. 11. London, HMSO.

Raw, M., McNeill, A., and West, R. (1998). Smoking cessation guidelines for health professionals: a guide to effective smoking cessation interventions for the health care system. *Thorax* Suppl., **5**, 1–38.

Smith, S., Warnakulasuriya, K., Feyerabend, C., *et al.* (1998). A smoking cessation programme conducted through dental practices in the UK. *British Dental Journal*, **185**, 299–303.

Speight, P., Downer, M., and Zakrzewska, J. (ed.) (1993). Screening for oral cancer and precancer: report of a UK working group. *Community Dental Health*, **10** (Suppl. 1), 1–89.

Stell, P. and McCormick, M. (1985) Cancer of the head and neck: are we doing any better? *Lancet*, **11**, 1127.

The Brewers Society (1999). *Statistical Handbook*, London, Brewers Society.

Thomas, M., Walker, A., Wilmot, A., and Bennet, N. (1998). *Office for National Statistics. Living in Britain: results from the 1996 General Household Survey*. London, The Stationery Office.

Watt, R. and Robinson, M. (1999). *Helping smokers to stop: a guide for the dental team*. London, Health Education Authority.

Watt, R., Johnson, N., and Warnakulasuriya, K. (2000). Action on smoking – opportunities for the dental team. *British Dental Journal*, **189**, 357–60.

WHO (World Health Organization) (1986). *The Ottawa Charter for Health Promotion*. Health Promotion 1. iii–v. Geneva, WHO.

FURTHER READING

Cancer Research Campaign (2000). *CRC CancerStats: Oral – UK*. London, Cancer Research Campaign.

Speight, P., Downer, M., and Zakrzewska, J. (ed.) (1993). Screening for oral cancer and precancer: report of a UK working group. *Community Dental Health*, **10** (Suppl. 1), 1–89.

Watt, R. and Robinson, M. (1999). *Helping smokers to stop: a guide for the dental team*. London, Health Education Authority.

West, R., McNeill, A., and Raw, M. (2000). Smoking cessation guidelines for health professionals: an update. *Thorax*, **55**, 987–99.

16 Public health approaches to the prevention of traumatic dental injuries

CONTENTS

By the end of this chapter you should be able to:

- Describe the key epidemiological data on traumatic dental injuries.
- Identify the main aetiological factors in traumatic dental injuries.
- Critically assess preventive approaches in traumatic dental injuries.
- Present public health approaches to the prevention of traumatic dental injuries.

This chapter links with:
- Introduction to the principles of public health (Chapter 1).
- Public health approaches to prevention (Chapter 4).
- Overview of epidemiology (Chapter 5).
- Principles of oral health promotion (Chapter 9).

INTRODUCTION

Injuries are a major cause of morbidity and mortality in both developed and developing countries around the world. The public health significance of injuries (see Box 16.1) has been recognized in the UK and is now one of the priority target areas in, for example the English Public Health strategy (Department of Health 1999).

In dentistry increasing clinical and public health interest has focused on the issue of traumatic dental injury. This chapter will present an overview of the epidemiology of traumatic dental injury. The impact of the condition will be highlighted and the key aetiological factors identified. A critical appraisal of treatment and preventive approaches will be presented and an alternative public health approach will be outlined.

Box 16.1 Public health impact of injuries

- Injuries claim over 10 000 lives per year in the UK.
- Nearly one-third of deaths among 15–24-year-olds are due to road traffic accidents.
- Every year more than 3000 people aged over 65 years die from falls.
- Children under 15 years from unskilled families are five times more likely to die from injury than those from professional families
- The NHS spends £1.6 billion every year to treat injury cases.

(Department of Health 1999)

EPIDEMIOLOGY OF TRAUMATIC DENTAL INJURIES

Data on the extent and severity of dental injuries is rather limited in comparison to the amount of information available in relation to dental caries and periodontal diseases. In the UK the national children's dental survey has collected data on dental injury since 1973, and other local surveys have also collected information. Direct comparisons of the findings from different studies are very difficult due to the variation in methods used and the sampling procedures. For example, the diagnostic criteria used in the 1983 and 1993 national child dental surveys (O'Brien 1994; Todd and Dodd 1985) was different than that used in the 1973 survey (Todd 1975).

DISCUSSION POINTS

Several different indices have been developed to assess the prevalence of dental injuries. What difficulties may be associated with the measurement of dental injuries?

Data from the most recent national UK child dental survey indicate an overall prevalence of dental injuries of 17% (O'Brien 1994). Variation across the UK was evident; for example, at 14 years children living in England had fewer dental injuries (15%) than children in Northern Ireland (18%), Wales (20%), and Scotland (23%).

Two large local surveys in deprived locations have identified a higher prevalence of dental injury than the national UK survey. A study of 11–14-year-olds in Bury and Salford in the north west of England reported a prevalence of 34.4% (Hamilton *et al.* 1997). A recent survey in the east end of London identified the prevalence of dental injuries in a sample of 14-year-olds as 23.7% (Marcenes and Murray 2001). A consistent finding in most surveys is that more boys than girls experience dental injury and that the peak age for this condition is early adolescence.

IMPACT OF CONDITION

Injuries to teeth vary greatly in severity, from minor enamel cracks to tooth fracture or luxation. The impact of the condition on the individual affected will therefore also vary greatly.

DISCUSSION POINTS

Outline the range of possible impacts dental injury may have on an individual's quality of life.

Describe the potential impact of dental injuries on the wider society.

With a substantial decline in caries in most developed countries, the costs of treating dental injury may soon equal that of caries. Although it is very difficult to calculate exact costings for different elements of dental care, those for the management and care of dental injuries are substantial due to the complexity and long-term nature of treatments. Research from Scandinavia in the 1990s estimated a cost of US$3.2–3.5 million per million subjects (Andreasen and Andreasen 1990, 1997). At a national UK level, the costs would therefore be very significant; about US$179–196 million, calculated at 1990s prices.

AETIOLOGY

Traumatic dental injuries are caused by a complex array of factors (Box 16.2). As in many other areas of dentistry, the individual clinical aetiological factors have tended to be highlighted as the most important. Incisal protrusion, increased overjet, and inadequate lip coverage are all important clinical risk factors but it is essential that the social, economic, and environmental determinants are also recognized as being fundamentally important. A strong social class gradient exists for childhood deaths caused by injury (Department of Health 1999), although the link between dental trauma and deprivation has not been thoroughly investigated. However, the surveys from deprived areas in the north-west of England and the east end of London have shown far higher rates of dental injuries than the national figures (Hamilton *et al.* 1997; Marcenes and Murray 2001). The study in London identified a greater risk of dental injury for subjects living in overcrowded households (Marcenes and Murray 2001).

Box 16.2 Risk factors for dental injuries

Clinical
- Incisal protrusion
- Increased overjet (> 6 mm)
- Inadequate lip coverage

Social/environmental
- Contact sports.
- Violence.
- Deprivation – overcrowding.
- Falls.
- Traffic and bicycle accidents.
- Poor environments.

LIMITATIONS OF TREATMENT AND PREVENTIVE OPTIONS

The clinical approach to the treatment and prevention of traumatic dental injuries is limited (see Box 16.3), and provides a good example of the shortcomings of clinical dentistry when no complementary public health approach is adopted. Orthodontics, restoring traumatized teeth, and the provision of mouth guards for contact sports, the traditional approaches to treatment and prevention, will only have a limited effect on the problem of dental injury.

Box 16.3 Limitations of the clinical approach to prevention and treatment of dental injuries

- High costs of treatment.
- Clinical time.
- Lack of clinical expertise.
- Poor treatment outcomes.
- Inequitable access to treatment and care.
- Palliative: fundamental causes of condition are not addressed.

The most recent national children's dental survey showed that nearly 60% of damaged incisors were in need of restorative treatment (O'Brien 1994). As mentioned previously, the costs of providing appropriate treatment for dental trauma cases would be substantial, assuming of course that clinicians in primary dental care have the skill and experience to successfully treat cases that present to them. It is apparent that, in addition to high-quality clinical care, greater emphasis needs to be placed upon reducing the number of cases that occur. This requires a public health approach which directs attention at changing the underlying conditions and causes of the problem.

PUBLIC HEALTH AGENDA

Earlier chapters have outlined public health approaches to the prevention of caries, periodontal disease, and oral cancer. As broadly similar recommendations have been made for these conditions there is little point in repeating them again for dental injury. Instead, in the following box a series of questions are presented. Discussing and answering these points will be a useful means of revising the principles outlined in the earlier chapters.

DISCUSSION POINTS

In a very deprived area of east London the prevalence of traumatic dental injury amongst teenagers is higher than the average UK figure. As a public health dentist working in that area you are required to develop a public health strategy to combat this problem. Consider the following points.

- What factors within the area may be responsible for the high prevalence of dental injury?
- Describe the different agencies, sectors, and organizations that you would need to work with to successfully tackle this problem.
- Outline what actions you would recommend to reduce the prevalence of dental injury within the school population.
- How would you evaluate your recommended actions?

CONCLUSION

Available epidemiological evidence indicates that traumatic dental injury is a significant public health problem. Conventional preventive and treatment approaches are unlikely to be successful unless a complementary public health strategy is adopted. Effective public health action will require collaborative working across sectors to alter the social, economic, and environmental conditions that are linked to dental injury.

REFERENCES

Andreasen, J. and Andreasen, F. (1990). Dental traumatology: quo vadis. *Endodontic and Dental Traumatology*, **6**, 160–9.

Andreasen, J. and Andreasen, F. (1997). Dental trauma. In *Community oral health* (ed. C. Pine), pp. 94–9. Oxford, Wright.

Department of Health (1999). *Saving lives: our healthier nation*. London, The Stationery Office.

Hamilton, F., Hill, F., and Holloway, P. (1997). An investigation of dento-alveolar trauma and its treatment in an adolescent population. Part 1: The prevalence and incidence of injuries and the extent and adequacy of treatment received. *British Dental Journal*, **182**, 91–5.

Marcenes, W. and Murray, S. (2001). Social deprivation and traumatic dental injuries among 14-year-old schoolchildren in Newham, London. *Dental Traumatology*, **17**, 17–21.

O'Brien, M. (1994). *Children's dental health in the UK 1993*. London, The Stationery Office.

Todd, J. (1975). *Children's dental health in England and Wales 1973*. London, HMSO.

Todd, J. and Dodd, T. (1985). *Children's dental health in the UK 1983*. London, HMSO.

FURTHER READING

Andreasen, J. and Andreasen, F. (1994). *Textbook and color atlas of traumatic injuries to the teeth*. Copenhagen, Munksgaard.

4

Health services

17 Overview of health care systems

CONTENTS

By the end of this chapter you should be able to:

- Outline the range of factors that influence the development of health care systems.
- Describe the different components of a health care system.
- Outline criteria by which health care systems could be evaluated..

This chapter links with:
- Introduction to the principles of public health (Chapter 1).
- All the other chapters in this section (Chapters 18–24).

INTRODUCTION

Health care systems are complex organizations that are in a constant process of change and evolution. Dentistry is one very small component of the wider health care system, which is itself part of the overall social welfare system within society. Dentists, as health professionals, need to understand the basic elements of the health care system within which they are working. This chapter will present an overview of health care systems, and a more detailed account of various issues raised will be covered in Chapters 18–24.

BACKGROUND

Modern health care systems and the health professions providing care within them have a long history of evolution and development. Across the world different systems of health care have emerged, linked to the social and political changes within each country. Historically only the wealthy had access to doctors, but gradually systems of care developed for a wider range of groups in society, often due to concerns over political instability and the fitness of army recruits (Mays 1991).

The nature of modern health care systems largely reflect the values and priorities of the societies in which they have developed. In the US a largely privately funded and organized health system operates, based upon the notion of individual responsibilities. In total contrast, health services in countries such as Cuba or China are state controlled and publicly funded. These systems are based upon a concept of collective benefit. Later in this chapter details will be presented of the different ways in which health care can be organized and delivered.

> **Box 17.1** Factors influencing health care systems
>
> - Changing patterns of disease.
> - Socio-demographic changes.
> - Public demands and expectations.
> - Professional development.
> - High technology.
> - International affairs – globalization.
> - Government health policy and reform programmes.

FACTORS INFLUENCING DEVELOPMENT OF MODERN HEALTH CARE SYSTEMS

A host of complex and inter-related factors influence how health care systems develop and change. Box 17.1 presents a summary of some of the key factors.

Enormous changes have taken place in the diseases that present to health professionals. In the nineteenth century acute infectious conditions were the greatest problems facing health systems in the Westernized world, with infectious disease hospitals and sanatoriums being built to care for people who survived the initial infection. Today chronic health conditions are the major challenge facing modern medicine. Conditions such as heart disease, mental illness, arthritis, and diabetes affect a large proportion of the population, often for many years. Health services are now required to provide long-term care and support for people affected by these conditions to improve their quality of life and maintain their independence.

Socio-demographic shifts in the population have occurred and continue to do so. For example, increasing numbers of very old people are living longer and requiring support and care. Ethnic and cultural diversity is a feature of modern British society. Appropriate services therefore need to be provided for different groups in the community.

DISCUSSION POINTS

What effect would the increasing numbers of very old people who are now living in the UK have on the NHS?

The public is now far more aware and knowledgeable about health issues, principally through the media's obsession with health matters, and increasingly expect and demand services to meet their needs. The growth of consumerism, in which health service users are now more empowered to challenge health professionals, places different demands on the provision and delivery of care.

Historically doctors and nurses, and to a lesser extent dentists, were the only professions that worked in health services. In recent decades there has been a great expansion in the range and diversity of health professions. Increasingly a team approach to care is being developed, in which different professionals contribute their particular skill and expertise. Specialization is also a feature of modern health services. A range of medical and dental specialities have developed over the years, which has implications for both professional training and service delivery.

DISCUSSION POINTS

List all the health professionals that work in the NHS.
Describe what different teams of professionals work together in the health service.

Modern medicine and dentistry rely heavily on high technology in terms of treatments, equipment, materials, and diagnostic procedures. Technology is generally expensive and requires technical support and maintenance. The pharmaceutical industry is dominated by multi-national corporations who wield enormous power and influence over national governments and health policy decisions.

A final major influence over how health care systems have developed, and indeed are constantly evolving, is the effect of changing political priorities and health policy developments. In the last 30 years the NHS has undergone a whole series of reviews and reform programmes. Many of these reforms have been driven by political dogma, whereas others were in accordance with international consensus on health services developments.

COMPONENTS OF HEALTH CARE SYSTEMS

To acquire a basic understanding of complex health care systems it is helpful to separate out and describe the different components of the system. Gift *et al.* (1997) have suggested the following approach:

- Structure: how is the system organized?
- Functions: what does the system aim to achieve?
- Personnel: who works in the system?
- Funding: how is the system funded?
- Reimbursement: how are the health professionals paid?
- Target population: who does the system provide care for?

Structure

The organization and structure is one of the most complex and dynamic components of the system. However, three basic levels of care often exist within a system:

- *Primary*: local general and routine services, which are the first point of contact between the public and the system; for example, general practitioners, pharmacists, general dental practitioners.
- *Secondary*: specialist services provided in hospital settings; for example, district general hospital.
- *Tertiary*: centres of clinical excellence, which are often teaching and research institutions; for example, university hospitals.

In the NHS the primary care sector, as the first point of contact with the system, acts as the 'gatekeeper' to the secondary and tertiary sectors. In some other systems individuals can directly access specialist services without the need for any referral.

DISCUSSION POINTS

What are the advantages and disadvantages of the gatekeeper system of referral?

Health services can be provided in a range of different settings (see Box 17.2), although frequently the locations of services do not match the population's health needs. In other words, health services are often located in areas where the needs are low, but in areas where the needs are greatest, few services are found, the so-called 'inverse care law' (Tudor Hart 1971).

Functions

Traditionally, health services following the medical model have aimed at curing disease in sick patients. It is now increasingly recognized, however, that few cures or 'magic bullets' exist, and indeed many treatments have

---

Box 17.2 Settings for health service delivery

- Hospitals
- Health centres and clinics
- General practices
- Dental surgeries
- Direct access centres
- Mobile surgeries
- Domiciliary care
- Workplace
- Pharmacists' premises

only limited effectiveness (Cochrane 1972). Instead, a core function of medicine is to provide care and support for individuals suffering from chronic conditions to improve their quality of life (McKeown 1979).

Although the provision of treatments is the dominant activity within health services, other functions are also performed to a lesser extent. These include:
- preventive advice to patients;
- health promotion within the community;
- epidemiological surveying;
- population screening;
- research;
- quality assurance and review;
- training;
- personnel.

Personnel

A range of different personnel are employed within health services; indeed, the NHS is now the largest employer in Western Europe. Although different health professions supply clinical care to patients, an array of technical, administrative, and support staff provide an essential service to the system. Many of these posts are very poorly paid, and the working conditions are frequently far from ideal.

What distinguishes health professionals from the other staff employed within health services? Friedson (1970) has developed a core set of defining characteristics of the professions:
- Tasks are highly skilled and require specialized knowledge.
- Registration provides a monopoly of their field of work.
- Professions have enjoyed considerable autonomy and self-regulation.
- A code of ethical practice prevents malpractice and exploitation of the public.
- Social status and financial rewards place the professions firmly within the middle classes.

Funding

Spending on health services has been rising steadily in most industrialized countries for many years. Indeed the escalating costs of funding health services has become a major concern for many governments and has been one of the main motivations for reforming the systems. The main reasons for the increasing costs of the NHS are:
1. Health care inflation has exceeded the general rate of inflation.
2. Numbers of staff employed in the system have risen sharply.
3. Demands on the system have steadily increased with more people presenting for care.
4. The proportion of people over 75 years has more than doubled in the last 50 years.

Table 17.1 Health care expenditure and gross domestic product 1997

	GDP per person (£)	Health care expenditure per person (£)			% of GDP
		Private	Public	Total	
UK	13301	138	752	889	6.7
EU average	13580	244	839	1083	7.9
USA	17822	1331	1165	2497	14.0
Switzerland	21546	659	1529	2188	10.2

In 1999 the total cost of the NHS was £51 billion. This figure is low compared to most other Western countries (Table 17.1).

The basic sources of funding for health services are:

- Taxation: either general taxes or specified health tax.
- Insurance: paid by individuals and/or employers.
- Direct payment from individuals.

Reimbursement systems

A range of different methods have been developed to reimburse health professionals for their services. Systems of reimbursement can become very complex when a mixture of different methods of payment are utilized. Essentially there are four basic systems of payment:

- Fee for item: practitioners are paid a fee for each item of work they provide.
- Capitation: payment is based upon the numbers of patients the practitioner has registered under their care.
- Salary: employers pay an annual income for the services provided by practitioners.
- Sessional arrangements: a set fee is agreed in a contract between employer and practitioner.

The advantages and disadvantages of the different options are discussed in Chapter 19.

Target population

Universal and fair access for the whole population was a founding principle of the NHS. In reality, access, and indeed the quality of services obtained, are not equal across society. Many marginalized and disadvantaged groups face numerous obstacles and barriers to access services, and the quality of care they receive once they enter the system is often inadequate (Benzeval *et al.* 1995).

DISCUSSION POINTS

What groups in society may have difficulty accessing the NHS?

How could these problems be addressed?

Based upon an assessment of particular needs or characteristics of potential users, different services within the system may also be targeted at groups within the population. Box 17.3 lists a range of potential target groups.

Box 17.3 Target population groups

- Infants and nursing mothers; for example, mother and baby groups.
- Pregnant women; for example, antenatal groups.
- Children and adolescents; for example, schools and colleges.
- Adults; for example, workplace.
- Older people; for example, day centres.
- Disabled groups; for example, people with mental illness.
- Disadvantaged groups; for example, homeless people.

WHAT IS A GOOD HEALTH CARE SYSTEM?

The British NHS, just like other health care systems around the world, has certain strengths and weaknesses. No system is perfect in all respects.

DISCUSSION POINTS

Based upon your general knowledge and any personal experiences, what do you consider are the strengths of the NHS?

In your opinion what are the weaknesses of the NHS?

One needs certain criteria to reach an informed judgement about whether a health system is good or not. From a public health perspective it is important that any assessment considers not only the views of the health professions but also includes a range of opinions from the different stakeholders in the system. Therefore the views of the general public, users of the services, health service managers, health professionals, and the government all need to be considered.

Maxwell (1984) has developed a useful set of criteria to evaluate the quality of a health care system:

- Effectiveness: do the treatments and care provided in the system produce desired outcomes and benefits?

- Efficiency: how well are the resources used within the system?
- Accessibility: can individuals in need use and benefit from the system?
- Equity: does the service provide a fair system for accessing care and are the outcomes of use equal across groups of users?
- Social acceptability: does the service strive to accommodate the characteristics and expectations of diverse social groups across society?
- Relevance to need: is there a good match between the needs of the population and the services offered?

CONCLUSIONS

Health care systems are large and complex organizations. Although oral health and dentistry are a very small part of the larger system, it is important that dental professionals have a basic understanding of the factors influencing service developments and the different components of the system. This chapter has provided an overview of health care systems. A more detailed account will now be provided of the NHS and in particular dental services in the UK.

REFERENCES

Benzeval, M., Judge, K., and Whitehead, M. (1995). *Tackling inequalities in health: an agenda for action*. London, Kings Fund.

Cochrane, A. (1972). *Effectiveness and efficiency*. London, Nuffield Provincial Hospital Trust.

Freidson, E. (1970). *Profession of medicine*. New York, Dodds, Mead.

Gift, H., Andersen, R., and Chen, M. (1997). The principles of organisation and models of delivery of oral health care. In *Community oral health* (ed. C. Pine), pp. 252–266. Oxford, Wright.

Hart, J. (1971). The inverse care law. *Lancet*, **i**, 405–12.

McKeown, T. (1979). *The role of medicine*. Oxford, Basil Blackwell.

Maxwell, R. (1984). Quality assessment in health. *British Medical Journal*, **288**, 1470–2.

Mays, N. (1991). Origins and development of the National Health Service. In *Sociology as applied to medicine*, 3rd edn (ed. G. Scambler), pp. 185–211. London, Baillière Tindall.

FURTHER READING

Pine, C. (ed.) (1997). *Community oral health*. Oxford, Wright.

18 The structure of the NHS in the UK

CONTENTS

By the end of this chapter you should be able to:

- Describe the general principles by which health care services are funded and organized in the UK.
- Understand the factors that have influenced the delivery of health care over the last 50 years.
- Describe the major problems faced by health services.
- Describe the main ways in which services are delivered.

This chapter links with:
- Overview of health care systems (Chapter 17).
- Planning dental services (Chapter 21).
- The structure of dental services in the UK (Chapter 19).

INTRODUCTION

The National Health Service was formed at the end of the Second World War. Its structure remained very stable until the 1970s, when it faced its first reform, and since then it has been constantly changing. The NHS has almost never taken a typical theoretical planning approach but rather has evolved because of a wide range of factors and influences. These include powerful professions, rationing of services, economic theory (market forces and the internal market), and changing governments with widely varying political views. The history of the service and the lessons of the past can inform the present and how the future may look.

This chapter outlines the major influences at work over the decades, describing the major problems faced by the health service and giving an overview of the ways in which clinical services are currently delivered. It will not give a detailed description of the structure of the health service, because by the time the book is published it is likely to be out of date! The current structure of the health service in each of the four countries of the UK will be available on this book's website, and updated as changes occur.

The original purpose of the health service was to alter the health of the nation by providing free and universal access to health care. However, it became apparent very quickly after the NHS's inception that it was not going to be possible to provide all the health care that was wanted and the service very quickly changed from having the belief that it could improve the nation's health into one which was trying to help people benefit from health care.

OUTLINE OF THE STRUCTURE

The history of the NHS ties in closely with that of the development of a welfare policy for this country and the type and policies of government. Following the Second World War the welfare policy of the country was based around five principles, for improving:
- education
- housing
- health
- pension
- squalor.

The emphasis on each of these has changed throughout the last 50 years. At the start all elements were of equal importance, but now more attention is placed upon health and education and less on pensions and housing. This reflects the changing views of each successive government and also public opinion.

FUNDING

The NHS is funded primarily by general taxation, free at the point of delivery, but there are some notable exceptions to this. In particular, dental services delivered through the General Dental Services are subject to patient co-payments (usually called 'charges'). However, this should not be viewed as being the total expenditure upon health. Individuals pay towards direct health costs in the private sector as well as by contributing to insurance or pre-payment plans, and this is particularly common in dentistry. This remains a relatively small part of the budget but is considered by some to be growing. In addition to this expenditure on 'formal' health care, people buy other health care items for use in the home.

The national budget is set each year and depends on the following factors:
- The level of spending from previous years – the 'historical' budget.
- The desired level of public expenditure, which in turn depends on the Public Spending Borrowing Requirement, the rates of taxation, and the general state of the economy, which will affect the government's income.
- The priorities as set by government.

Although the budget is agreed each year in a series of negotiations between the Treasury and those departments known as 'the high spenders' – education and health – the changes are usually only marginal. It is extremely difficult to reduce the budget from the previous year's expenditure. In most years the increase in expenditure is greater than that required by inflation but there are two reasons why this is often considered to be insufficient. Firstly, the rate of inflation in the health sector is higher than the general rate, and secondly the introduction of new techniques and drugs can increase the costs overall.

The expenditure on health is routed through the Department of Health (for England) and the three appropriate bodies in the other constituent countries (Scottish Executive, National Assembly for Wales, and Northern Irish Assembly). Money is distributed broadly on a population basis to geographical areas. Adjustments are made for issues such as rural areas. Some areas of the country, particularly those with teaching hospitals or major tertiary services, have received more funding than would be expected on the basis of their population. A series of schemes, since 1974, have attempted to alter the historical funding which gave these areas proportionately higher levels of resources but although some changes have resulted these have been very small.

MAJOR INFLUENCES OVER LAST 50 YEARS

The 1940s saw the emergence of professionalism and, at the end of the decade, the creation of the NHS. Dentistry was included, although there was much unmet need and dentists soon had far more work than had been anticipated. There was a paternalistic attitude to health care: the professions knew what was best for their patients.

The 1950s saw the NHS established as a social model based on equity and universal access, and it remained dominated by the professions. Even at this early stage in its development it was clear that there were not enough resources to fund all demands. Patient charges were introduced in 1951 for dentistry. As Gelbier (1994) said, 'Health care rationing by charge had been introduced.'

The 1960s continued in much the same way as the 1950s, except that financial problems were starting to become apparent within the UK and the pressure on the NHS to contain costs started to become more pronounced.

The 1970s saw the first reform of the NHS, with the introduction of a very complex structure based upon the concept of consensus management. There was representation of many groups but no professional managers were included at that time. They were known as administrators. For the first time concepts such as planning health services became important and this was encouraged by the realization that services were unequally distributed and that there was a need to attempt to redistribute them. The Black Report, published very quietly in 1980, demonstrated that 30 years' health care free at the point of delivery had not solved the problem of health inequalities, which persisted and in some places had become worse. There was a fiscal crisis caused, in part, by oil prices and rationing in the health service became more pronounced. By the end of the decade financial cuts were becoming apparent.

In the 1980s reforms became more frequent. Firstly, one tier of management was removed and then the concept of 'general management' was introduced. However, this was limited in that management was responsible for the financial control while clinical standards remained totally within the remit of the professionals. There was a major emphasis on cost-effectiveness which became almost synonymous with the cheapest being best. The political atmosphere meant that concepts such as 'society' did not exist, and it was considered preferable for people to have total responsibility for themselves.

Other very major trends started which were to develop further in the 1990s. 'Care in the Community' legislation meant that large numbers of long-stay hospitals for psychiatric illness and for people with learning disabilities were closed. Government policy was to care for as many people as possible within the community, but there was dispute as to whether enough money was transferred to care appropriately for these people.

Within the professions specialization evolved rapidly. The development of evidence-based care started, although it was not yet called that. Consumerism increased in importance, but more importantly the professions started to be criticized. Rationing became explicit – it was not possible to deliver all that was wanted. In the main this was controlled through waiting lists although some treatments were not available.

The 1990s saw a continuation of all the themes from the 1980s, combined with the most major reform since its inception. Two functions were identified: the estimation of need and planning of health care; and the provision of health care. Responsibilities for these functions were divided: health authorities assumed the function of 'commissioning' health care while trusts and the contractor professions 'provided' health care. The concept of market forces briefly entered the health service although by the end of the decade this had gone.

The professions continued to develop, with the introduction of clinical audit: clinical effectiveness became important. Cheapest was no longer best but rather the intervention that provided the best outcome for the best price was preferred.

The building of new hospitals started to become financed through agreements with private companies (Private Financial Initiatives).

A number of scandals arose in the health service, which resulted in the independence of the professions being criticized. These led to the introduction of 'clinical governance', a system of total quality assurance where the chief executive of the organization now had responsibility for clinical as well as financial matters.

The commissioning of health care was reviewed at the end of the decade, when it was decided that this role should be returned to those who were considered to understand the needs best – the primary care practitioners.

The change of government at the end of the decade to the first Labour government in many years led to a massive alteration in policy. Public health was considered to be very important, and documents were published (Department of Health 1998b; Scottish Office 1998; Welsh Office 1998b)

Box 18.1 Aims of 1998 reforms

- Remove competition from the health service.
- Encourage interdisciplinary functioning, particularly including working with other agencies, notably local authorities, to improve health. This acknowledges a different approach to the causes of ill health. It shows that policy in central government has moved away from a purely medical model.
- The new system will evolve towards increasing the role of the general medical practitioner in deciding what health care is required. This will be done through developing groups of general medical practices working together, initially with health authorities, to decide what care is required. The exact system varies between countries: in Wales they will be co-terminous with local authorities while in England they will serve groups of approximately 100 000 people.

---

which highlighted the very real health inequalities that existed in society. Health services were to work closely with other bodies, particularly local authorities, to alter the determinants of health.

In 1999 elections resulted in the creation of new parliaments and assemblies in the countries as a result of the devolution of power from Westminster. These bodies will have, as major responsibilities, health and education. It is possible that each of the four countries of the UK will develop different health policies, and even that the services provided will be different.

The new century brought the promise of a review of publicly funded services, with the role of private finance to be investigated. The bodies ruling the professions were subject to reform in order to increase the public's input into them. The government has promised to put the decision-making powers back into the hands of primary care providers.

WHICH DIRECTION?

The future of the health service is difficult to predict, but the influences that are currently occurring suggest that it will have to incorporate the following characteristics.

- It will be responsive to needs.
- It will be flexible.
- It will be responsive to consumer demands.
- It will be evidence-based.
- Planning and decisions will be made at a local level.
- It will be more integrated with other public services, particularly education and local authorities.
- It will have a team approach, with consideration given to skill mix but not just the professionals.

Box 18.2 The aims of NICE

- To improve continually the overall standards of clinical care.
- To reduce unacceptable variations in clinical practice.
- To ensure the best use of resources so that patients receive the greatest benefit.

(Welsh Office 1998a)

- It will be more of a partnership.
- The government of the day and its political view.

Clinical governance

A very important concept was introduced in the 1999 health service reorganization: the drive for quality improvement in the new NHS through a process known as clinical governance. It is important because for 'the first time, all health organizations will have a statutory duty to seek quality improvement through clinical governance' (Scally and Donaldson 1998). This process means that quality improvement is to be combined with financial management, and overall responsibility for this will rest with the chief executive of the health authority and of the trusts. Independent contractors such as general dental practitioners are also included in the system. The exact structures under which this will be achieved are developing slowly.

Two major new bodies have been set up and these are the National Institute for Clinical Excellence (NICE) and the Commission for Health Improvement (CHI).

NICE's main role is to identify techniques and therapies that need to be appraised. NICE looks at the clinical and cost-effectiveness evidence to produce guidelines. It also has a role in disseminating the results of its work. In essence, NICE examines developing and existing techniques and therapies to see if they work and how much they cost. It then decides whether these therapies and techniques should be undertaken within the NHS. The effect of this is that NICE has already recommended against some treatment; for example, the prophylactic removal of third molar teeth.

COMMISSIONING OF HEALTH SERVICES

Within the NHS health services are planned and provided within an overall budget. The health service has two functions. One function is that of commissioning health care, the process of deciding what health care should be provided. Not all hospitals provide, for example, cardio-thoracic surgery. There are a variety of factors which should be considered when deciding what should be provided, including epidemiology of the disease, need and demand for care, effectiveness of known treatments, effectiveness of treat-

---

Box 18.3 The core functions of CHI

- Provide national leadership to develop and disseminate clinical governance principles.
- Independently scrutinize local clinical governance arrangements to support, promote, and deliver high-quality services, through a rolling programme of local reviews of service providers.
- Undertake a programme of service reviews to monitor national implementation of National Service Frameworks, and review progress locally on implementation of these frameworks and NICE guidance.
- Help the NHS identify and tackle serious or persistent clinical problems. The commission will have the capacity for rapid investigation and intervention to help put these right.
- Over time, to increasingly take on responsibility for overseeing and assisting with external incident inquiries.

(Department of Health 1998a; Welsh Office 1998a)

---

ment centres, need for locally provided services, and availability of resources.

DISCUSSION POINTS

What other factors would you include as being important in deciding whether or not a service should be provided? What priority would you give to each factor? Are there any factors that are included that you think should be ignored? Why?

The health authorities have a major role in deciding what services should be commissioned and how resources should be used. However, there is an increasing role for bodies which are constituted slightly differently in each of the UK's constituent countries. These are the primary care trusts (PCTs) in England, the local health groups (LHGs) in Wales, the local health care co-operatives (LHCCs) in Scotland, and the health trusts in Northern Ireland. Although the constitution is different in each area, they share a similar principle: that decisions should be made by those with local knowledge and that general practitioners should be involved in making these decisions. Other health care professionals are also involved in these groups, including nurses. In Wales a dentist is on the LHG and is involved in the decision-making. However, this is not the case in England where oral health advisory groups (OHAGs) are encouraged in all areas where they provide information to the PCTs. In England the PCTs serve populations of various sizes, while in Wales LHGs are co-terminous with local authorities and are therefore much larger. These groups have been allocated the entire budget for health care in their area and are expected to decide how to spend it. The practice of giving the general medical practitioner a leading role in the commissioning of health care is seen as important because they are considered to have the necessary local knowledge to decide what is required.

> **DISCUSSION POINTS**
>
> What aspects of the locality may general practitioners know very well, and what aspects may they know less well? What additional skills and help may they need?

General practitioners have always had a very important role in the NHS because they are the 'gatekeepers' to secondary health care. This means that it is not possible for someone to see a consultant in a hospital unless a general practitioner makes a referral. Although common in the UK, this is not so in Europe where it is possible to go directly to any specialist that is wanted.

> **DISCUSSION POINTS**
>
> What are the advantages and disadvantages of being able to go to a specialist directly? You need to look at this both from both the individual's and the health care system's points of view.

One aspect of the commissioning of health care services that may be more difficult is for those services that are planned on a larger population basis than that served by a group of general medical practices. Certain services such as those for cancer are planned on a regional basis because of issues surrounding quality. Where dentistry will fit into this scheme is not yet clear.

PROBLEMS AND CHALLENGES

Problems facing all public services

All services funded through a welfare policy are faced with the same major problem. They need to justify their existence. Why should the state provide health care for its citizens through taxation? Would it not be better if each person paid for their own medical care as and when they needed it?

The challenge is therefore to deliver their service to a measurable standard related to evidence-based care.

Problems and challenges facing health care

This chapter concentrates on those that affect the whole of the country at the moment: the macro problems. The micro problems are discussed elsewhere.

Treats demand rather than need

The NHS provides care to people who ask for help. Thus it treats demand for care rather than need for care. The effect of this is that the inappropriate care may be being delivered.

Increased expenditure although growth in real terms

Although the NHS budget is growing in real terms the required or wanted expenditure is growing at a faster rate. As such it is not possible to provide all health care that is wanted.

Conflict between cost of treatment and clinical effectiveness

Clinical effectiveness is important in ensuring that the most effective care is provided for a given condition. However, this does not mean that the cheapest treatment will be used and it may be that by altering therapies to those known to be more clinically effective, treatment costs will increase markedly. Clinical effectiveness also needs to result in disinvestment in those therapies that have been shown to have no worth, and thus lead to a release of resources. Decisions are going to be more difficult to make where the improved clinical benefit is only marginal but the cost is much greater. It is not known how these borderline decisions will be made.

Ageing population

Within the UK there is an ageing population: proportionately there are fewer younger people and more older people. This will have two important effects on the health service. Firstly, there will be more older people to care for, and it may be that there will be more chronic disease to treat, which will increase expenditure. However, there is evidence that the greatest expenditure on a person is during their last year of life, at whatever age that occurs. This may mean that the expected increased expenditure is likely to result simply because a greater proportion of the population are reaching the end of their natural life. Secondly, the fact that the population is ageing means that fewer people are entering the workforce. This may increase costs in the health sector if salaries have to increase to attract people to work in these areas.

Increase in inequalities

The health inequalities within the UK mean that there is a need for a reallocation of resources towards areas with poorer health, or towards actions that will differentially improve health in these areas. It is acknowledged that many of these activities may be outside the health sector. How this will alter funding is not known.

Care is rationed in some areas

The health care that is provided is decided by the commissioning bodies. There are no standards stating what services must be provided, which means that there can be variations between areas. Examples that have been discussed in the press include the provision of infertility treatment in different areas.

DISCUSSION POINTS

What are the implications of providing slightly different services in different areas? What are the advantages and disadvantages?

Health care is a political issue

Within the UK the main decisions regarding the funding and structure of health care are taken within government. Health is seen as an important issue that strongly influences the electorate's decision on who to vote for. Members of parliament are often approached by constituents to discuss problems within the health service, which means that locally based problems can have an extremely high public profile and solutions may be negotiated through the media.

DISCUSSION POINTS

What should the balance be between media access to all health care provision and ability to make decisions out of the media's eye?

HEALTH CARE DELIVERY IN THE UK

Primary care

Most health care is provided through primary care and access to secondary services is controlled through this route. The main section of the workforce working in primary care are independent contractors, doctors, dentists, pharmacists, and opticians, who are supported by their own employees. A second group are employees of the health service, which include groups such as health visitors, district nurses, and community dental service staff.

Independent contractors

The medical contract

The contract under which general practitioners are employed is based upon the principle of the number of patients registered with them. While this remains the major way in which they are paid, the contract has developed to include payment for achieving certain levels of immunization rates and other fee-for-item of service payments. Doctors also receive grants for their premises.

The dental contract

Dentistry has always been funded upon a different basis. General dental practitioners run a small business, and they are responsible for all their capital costs and staff costs. They are free to see as many or as few patients as they want and can determine the mix between private and NHS care. The dental contract basically pays dentists for the amount of work they undertake on a fee-for-item of payment. There is a small component for continuing care of patients, paid monthly. In general, if a general dental practitioner does not work he or she does not get paid.

Community health employees

District nurses provide nursing support for those at home on a day-to-day basis. With the increasing emphasis on early discharge from hospital they have a very important role as well as providing nursing care for those who are not able to care for themselves.

Health visitors provide health promotion advice and support to parents of those under 5 years.

Intermediate care

Within general practice the concept of intermediate care has developed. A general practitioner has special skills and expertise in a disease such as diabetes. He/she manages all the patients of the practice (and maybe neighbouring practices), thus relieving the secondary care service of a considerable volume of work. This is one area in which expansion is planned.

Secondary care

This is provided by consultants and other specialist-grade staff. It is almost entirely based in hospitals and, as has been said, the primary care practitioners are the gatekeepers to secondary care.

Tertiary care

Some services are provided on a regional or even national basis, and are known as tertiary services. One of the major problems with tertiary services is that they can be quite some distance from people's local health services. The concept of 'managed clinical networks', where various parts of the specialist care will be provided in different localities, is being developed.

Other sectors

It is very important to note the role of the social services, particularly in providing care and support for people with disabilities. The voluntary sector is important in such things as providing hospice care. The main area in which the private sector provides care is in the provision of nursing homes for the elderly.

CONCLUSIONS

The NHS is a highly complex organization that continues to evolve. It provides a very wide range of services, mainly free at point of delivery. In the future it aims to become more locally responsive and more integrated with other services. In the 1990s it finally acknowledged the need to deal with some of the determinants of health. It remains to be seen if it is possible to alter the direction of such a large organization.

REFERENCES

Black, D., Morris J. N., Smith, C., and Townsend, P. (ed.) (1980). *Inequalities in health: report of a research working group*. DHSS, London.
Department of Health (1998a). *First class service*. Health Service Circular 113/98.
Department of Health (1998b). *Our healthier nation*. London, The Stationery Office.
Gelbier, S. (1994). Where have we come from? In *Introduction to dental public health* (ed. M. Downer, S. Gelbier, and D. Gibbons), pp. 11–29. London, FDI World Dental Press.
Scally, G. and Donaldson, L. (1998). Clinical governance and the drive for quality improvement in the new NHS in England. *British Medical Journal*, 317, 61–5.
Scottish Office (1998). *Working together for a healthier Scotland*. London, The Stationery Office.
Welsh Office (1998a). *Quality care and clinical excellence*. London, The Stationery Office.
Welsh Office (1998b). *Better health, better Wales*. London, The Stationery Office.

19 The structure of dental services in the UK

CONTENTS

By the end of this chapter you should be able to:
- Describe how oral health care may be managed and organized.
- Describe the structure of oral health care in the UK.
- Describe the structure and features of the primary and secondary care sector in the provision of public sector dental care.
- Describe the structure and features of private dental care.
- Describe methods of remuneration for oral health personnel.
- Describe the role, training, and use of persons complementary to dentists in the provision of dental care.
- Describe the implications of current oral health policy for care delivery in the UK.

This chapter links with:
- Introduction to the principles of public health (Chapter 1).
- The structure of the NHS in the UK (Chapter 18).
- Planning dental services (Chapter 21).
- Problems with health services (Chapter 23).
- Dental organizations (Chapter 24).

INTRODUCTION

Health care systems evolve as part of the welfare structure of a society and will be influenced by the changes within that society. All health care systems have a number of core components: a method of raising revenues to finance the system, an organizational structure, a service component, and training arrangements. The provision of oral health care within the public sector in the UK has been shaped by developments to the National Health Service (NHS). The limited changes to the General Dental Services contract since its inception in 1948 has meant that the sector in which the majority of care provision occurs has hardly changed. With the exception of patient charges, what changes have occurred have done so without any real analysis of the issues of importance in dental care (House of Commons Health Committee 2001).

This chapter will briefly describe how oral health care may be managed and organized and how health workers may be remunerated. This will be followed by a short outline of the ways in which oral health care is provided in the UK, and an examination of the implications of current dental policy for the delivery of oral health care. A separate overview of persons complementary to dentistry is presented later in this chapter. The reform of the NHS is ongoing and readers should access this book's website to find current information (http://www.oup.org/edph).

FINANCING ORAL HEALTH CARE

Any oral health care system requires funding. In this section, options for the financing of oral health care are outlined, along with the advantages and disadvantages of each. There are two important issues to consider: the initial raising of revenue and how the funds are subsequently distributed.

Raising revenue

Funds for oral health care are in essence only derived from the public, either as a whole (collective funding) or from individuals. In a totally private system funds are derived directly from an individual to pay a dental worker without any third party involvement. However, this arrangement has built-in inequities: only those people who can afford to do so can buy care. As a result most societies intervene to ensure that certain sections of a society get subsidized treatment; for example, many countries provide free treatment for children and the elderly. This requires a redistribution of resources, and governments must raise funds through, for example, various forms of taxation. But for the moment let us remain with a purely private arrangement. Two routing models exist. In the first, as mentioned previously, no third party is involved. The patient pays the dentist directly for his or her treatment. However, a second model could exist, in which resources are allocated indirectly, for example by an insurance group who act on behalf of the consumer or patient in negotiating with the dental profession, either on an individual basis on with the profession as a whole.

Figure 19.1 illustrates these possible flows. The model that exists in the UK is in the main centred on routes 1 and 3, based on taxation, either direct or through national insurance contributions, and its subsequent allocation to various public funded services, including dentistry. In Germany, the arrangement is slightly different in that third party insurance groups are involved and a proportion of an individual's annual salary is allocated to health care. A third model operates in the United States under the guise of *managed care.* Individuals buy into a care plan which is organized by a health care company, which subsequently contracts with dentists to provide a level of care.

In route 2, the public pays the dentist directly for his or her services; this is a private arrangement. A third party may intervene to control pricing. For example, Dutch and Swedish adult dental care is now mostly in the private sector, but each year the profession negotiates the scale of fees with their government. Route 3 illustrates that once revenue has been raised, the resources will need to be distributed.

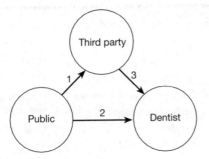

Fig. 19.1 Routing of funds for oral health care.

The subsequent distribution process for paying health care workers is illustrated in Fig. 19.2. There are again three mechanisms:
1. A purely private arrangement, where the state does not concern itself with the distributive aspects of the market.
2. The state pays the total cost through the allocation of resources raised by various mechanisms.
3. The co-payment models, where a contribution is made by the patient for the cost of his or her treatment.

Payment arrangements

Once the processes for the overall distribution mechanisms are identified, a number of different methods of remuneration exist. There are in essence four main ones, all aiming to reward a worker for achieving the prescribed goals: fee-per-item, a sessional fee, capitation, and salary. A mechanism that is often quoted as a fifth, but which in essence is simply a modification of the first and third, is performance-related pay. The sessional arrangement is

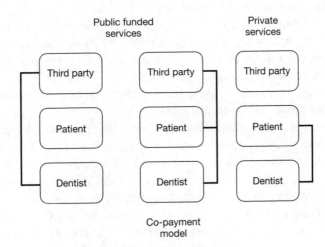

Fig. 19.2 Arrangement of distribution options.

Table 19.1 Main mechanisms for rewarding dental care workers

Mechanism	Advantages	Disadvantages
Fee-per–item	Good in areas of high need Reward for output Treatment focus Easy to measure	Potential for over-treatment Difficult to budget Little incentive for prevention
Sessional	Regular income Reward for output Minimize resource costs Option for special need groups	Adverse risk selection Under-treat patients Untried
Salaried	Administratively simple Facilitates budgeting Treatment not influenced by profit Other benefits: sick pay and maternity leave	Possible under-treatment Lack of financial incentives to work Requires extensive management structures
Capitation	Administratively simple Facilitates budgeting Reward linked to effort Treatment not influenced by profit	Adverse risk selection No knowledge of output Under-treatment of patients Payments 'unfair' in areas of high need compared to low need

a more flexible modification of a salaried system, although it can serve specific purposes that will be discussed later.

Under a fee-per-item arrangement, the reward is centred on rewarding according to the number of units produced. The more units produced, the greater the reward. Under capitation, the worker is paid a total fee to look after an individual. A salaried arrangement is simply an agreed sum of money, usually per annum, irrespective of the number of individuals under care or the number of items produced.

Table 19.1 lists the main advantages and disadvantages of each of the mechanisms. The two opposite ends of the spectrum are fee-per-item and capitation. In essence, when choosing between these two options one is either accepting a risk of over-treatment, which fee-per-item systems can encourage, or the risk of under-treatment that can occur under capitation. When choosing between the balance of the two the situation that exists at the time is critical. Where there is a shortage of labour and a large amount of work to be completed the fee-per-item is perhaps the most efficient choice.

However, where labour is in excess and the pool of work diminishing, capitation is a more sensible option. Irrespective of the problem to be solved, no single mechanism will provide the best solution. Nearly all care systems rely on both capitation and fee-per-item for payment of the majority of care and salaried arrangements for the minority. The latter include specialist services within the secondary care sector, that is, the hospital setting, and other groups where more conventional arrangements do not necessarily work well.

SUPPORT SYSTEMS

Irrespective of the payment system implemented, a number of prerequisites are required to maintain the arrangements. They can be divided into three: information systems, education systems, and probity systems.

Information systems

Information is required to assess three aspects of an oral health care system: the disease profiles, activity data, and management information. The goal of the reward (payment) system is to reduce the need for treatment. Workers should be paid commensurate with their contribution in achieving the reduction. In order to assess both the contribution and, more fundamentally, what is happening, a mechanism to collect disease data is required.

The most common standard is that adopted by the World Health Organization's (WHO) model. Data are collected on standard forms using set criteria. The data include caries levels, periodontal conditions, orthodontic data, and soft tissue information, although not every survey has to collect everything. The completed forms can be sent to the headquarters of WHO in Geneva for the analyses to be undertaken, and a summary report is returned to the researchers. These data are also in the public domain and are available at two web sites: caries data stored in Sweden (http://www.whocollab.od.mah.se/index.html), and periodontal data in Japan (http://www.dent.niigata-u.ac.jp/prevent/perio/contents.html).

Alternative data collection mechanisms have been introduced in the UK under the auspices of the British Association for the Study of Community Dentistry. These data are for 5-, 12-, and 14- year-olds, and have allowed a longitudinal database to be established, although only cross-sectional in nature (www.dhsru.ac.uk).

Many countries undertake national surveys to monitor disease levels. With the cost of training examiners and collecting the data, the justification for doing so needs to be made.

Education systems

Within any care system, the workforce needs to be trained to provide the appropriate level of care. Training is necessary at two levels: the initial arrangements, and the subsequent arrangements. The subsequent arrangements include the training necessary should one wish to become a specialist, or that simply necessary to keep up to date as part of continuing professional development requirements. Details of continuing professional development are available from the General Dental Council (http://www.gdc-uk.org). In addition to actual numbers of personnel, the other key area is the grade. One of the most contentious issues in oral health care delivery concerns skill mix and, in particular, to what extent professionals complementary to dentistry can undertake tasks currently carried out by dentists.

Ideally there should be a spectrum of skills, the particular mix of which is suited to the disease profile presented in a country. The rapid decline in disease in children and a growing more complex treatment need in older people produces a very different disease profile to say, one of 30 years ago. Matching the skills to the changes is very difficult. Clinical disease indicators influence the skills required, and new treatments and increased expectations all make it very difficult to identify the correct number of personnel with the appropriate skills. Even if the numbers could be identified, adjusting present training places takes time. For example, suppose tomorrow a government decided that more dentists were required. A dental school might need to be planned and built, which would take several years. Once the initial entrants started, it would still take 5 years for the graduates to enter the service.

This lead-in period is probably around 10 or so years and is further complicated by the fact that the working lifetime of a dentist is around 40 years. This creates a very inflexible system: one of the main reasons that alternative training programs using differing skill mixes are being examined. A second reason relates to costs; labour costs are the most expensive element of the care system. Therefore, in theory, mechanisms that allow care to be provided with a lower labour charge, for example by substituting dentists with school dental nurses, therapists, or hygienists, would allow more care for the same money or the same care for less money. This advantage has yet to be proven and current working practices mean that the savings may not be as great as forecast.

Probity systems

Probity is an assessment of the honest accountability of the activities of a system and consists of four components.
1. The accuracy of any fee claims. Whenever a claim is made under a system, the payer needs to make sure that what is being claimed for is valid. Has the filling been done or the scale and polish carried out?
2. Was the treatment carried out to a satisfactory standard? This requires both a clinical assessment and a reference standard. In the UK, one of the roles of the Dental Reference Service is to examine patients at random who have received care under the NHS and to grade the standard of

work. Other care systems also undertake such assessments, for example, the insurance companies in the USA.

3. In addition to a claim's validity and the standard of the treatment, the quality of the initial diagnosis and treatment planning is also important. The former is more difficult as patients tend to be seen once the treatment has been completed and a claim submitted. Nevertheless, the monitoring arrangements are such that abnormal patterns of treatment prescription by practitioners can be identified and explanations sought.

4. Finally, all systems will have limitations on the treatments provided and under what conditions they can be prescribed. These are described in the *terms of service*, the name given to the contract between the care provider and the paying agency. It may include such issues as limiting the total costs of a course of treatment before seeking prior approval in advance of undertaking the work, not being allowed to repeat work, making a claim for it before a certain date, and even what materials can be used.

The next section will describe the organizational structure, service components, methods of remuneration and training of personnel of oral health care in the UK.

ORAL HEALTH CARE IN THE UK

Oral health care provision in the UK occurs in both the public and the private sector. The public sector consists of three main sections: two branches of the primary care sector, the Community Dental Service and the far larger General Dental Service, and the secondary care sector, the Hospital Dental Service. Recently new reforms of local contracting have evolved and are known as the Personal Dental Services. Details can be found on the Department of Health website (http://www.doh.gov.uk/dental/). In addition, the armed forces provide their own dental service, the Dental Defence Agency, though the numbers involved are small. It has been suggested that the cost of the public health sector dental care is around £1674 million per year (Batchelor and Stirling 1998).

In addition to the public sector, treatment provision also occurs through the private sector. Payments for treatment under non-NHS arrangements are through a variety of mechanisms, including self-pay schemes, capitation, and insurance schemes. Recent estimates have calculated that the total spend on the private sector dentistry is around £926 million per year (Blackburn 1999).

THE PROVISION OF ORAL HEALTH CARE THROUGH THE PUBLIC SECTOR

The structure of public sector oral health care is illustrated in Fig. 19.3. The organization and structure of public funded oral care has been amended recently (National Health Service Executive 1997). The salaried dental services

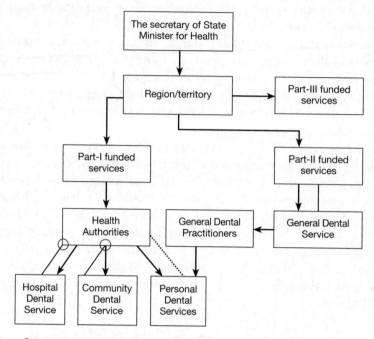

--------- Strict contractual arrangements around the cost and type of care provided

———O National agreed contract referring to registration, renumeration, and patient complaints

Fig. 19.3 The structure of public sector oral health care 2001. (From National Health Service Executive 1997.)

of the Hospital Dental Service and Community Dental Service continue to receive their funding from the health authority through *Part I*-funded services, a cash-limited budget. The General Dental Service is funded through a separate non-cash-limited budget, a *Part II*-funded service. The Personal Dental Services receives its funding from the health authority through both Part I- and Part II-funded services, the latter channelled through the General Dental Service. *Part III* - funded services are specialist tertiary services.

The General Dental Service: organizational structure and service component

The General Dental Service (GDS) was introduced as part of the NHS in 1948 and was free at the point of delivery. At the inception of the NHS there was a huge backlog of unmet treatment need and relatively few dentists. Dentists working within the NHS were independent contractors providing dental care to NHS patients on a fee-per-item basis. But by 1951 the ever increasing volume of dental treatment and associated escalating costs could not continue to be met by the NHS. Patient charges (co-payments) were introduced to make up for the short fall in funding (Gelbier 1994). Patients had a short-term contractual arrangement with their dentist, who would provide a course of treatment that would render them 'dentally fit'. While continuing care was not a feature of the arrangement, in reality many dentists built up a list of patients to whom they had an ongoing commitment (House of Commons Health Committee 2001).

DISCUSSION POINTS

How would you define the term 'dentally fit' as
- a dental patient?
- a dentist?
- the Minister for Health?

A complicated system for calculating the fee scale existed. A target annual gross income and a target annual net income were used to calculate what the average dentist would earn. Target annual gross income was based on the productivity of an 'average' dentist, while target annual net income was a hypothetical 'average' income after practice and other expenses were deducted. The fee scale was then modified in light of changes in target annual gross income. The structure of the GDS remained virtually unchanged until a new contract was introduced in 1990. Concerns had been expressed since the 1960s about the fee-per-item system of remuneration and the possible existence of over-treatment within the NHS. The objective behind the 1990 contract was to move dentists away from a short-term relationship with a patient to one in which continuing care existed. Under the contract patients were registered for a period of time, had access to out-of-hours emergency care, and greater continuity of care.

Dentists opposed the introduction of the new contract in 1990 amid fears that it would reduce their earnings. They actually increased their productivity that year by 8%. But the Dentists and Doctors Review Body, which recommends what the government should set as target annual gross income, underestimated the effects of the contractual changes and this lead to an overspend in the GDS of £19 million in the year 1991/92. In order to claw back the overspend, the government cut the fee scale by 23% (later reduced to 7%) for that following year (1992/3). This amounted to £12 000 per dentist for work already undertaken (Bradnock and Pine 1997). Dentists working within the GDS were furious and many actively moved away from providing NHS dental care. Before 1990, 8% of dental care was provided in private dental practice (Todd and Lader 1991), but by 1999 it was estimated that 24% of adult patients received some of their dental care through private arrangements (Anon 1999). The debacle over the fees prompted a wide-ranging enquiry into dental remuneration within the GDS. The government commissioned a report by Sir Kenneth Bloomfield (1992) that reviewed the current situation. Bloomfield made a number of observations

---

Box 19.1 Bloomfield Report: observations on the GDS

1. There was an absence of a dental strategy in all the constituent countries of the UK except Wales.
2. There was a lack of prioritization within the GDS.
3. Many of the problems within the GDS had been produced by the incentives and effects which occur in a fee-per-item system.
4. The notion of the average dentist was flawed.

(Bloomfield 1992)

---

about the GDS itself, which are reproduced in Box 19.1. The fee scale, as highlighted in the report, was felt not to have kept pace with inflation and dentists had increased their productivity to increase their earnings. The net effect, however, had been to increase the productivity of the 'average' dentist, but neither the target annual gross income nor target annual net income had kept pace. Thus the 'treadmill effect' was produced, with dentists producing more but earning less.

A national contract exists for the GDS and covers the registration of the patient, remuneration of the dentist, and other procedures, for example patient complaints. General Dental Practitioners (GDPs) operating within the GDS are self-employed contractors. They are not legally obliged to register patients. Contractual agreements do not specify details covering categories of patients seen, for example, the number of children, adults, or 'special need' patients, nor which items of treatment should be provided. In addition, since 1990, GDPs have been allowed to mix private and NHS dentistry.

Current remuneration arrangements

The overall budget for NHS GDS is based upon the average amount a full time dentist would be expected to earn (target annual gross income). The Dentists and Doctors Review Body reviews the work of the profession annually and decides a recommended remuneration for the average dentist. The government, having listened to the proposals made by the Dentists and Doctors Review Body, sets a level for that remuneration, given the overall budget for NHS dental care. The Dental Rates Study Group forecasts the average practice expenses and takes account of whether there was an over- or an underspend in the previous year's forecast. A fee scale is then produced which will provide an average net remuneration at the level agreed with government.

Currently, adult and child patients register with a GDP for 15 months and must re-attend within the 15-month period or registration 'lapses'. One-third of adults registered with the GDS are entitled to free dental treatment, including 18-year-olds in full time education, those on low income, job seekers, and pregnant women. The remainder of adults who are not eligible for free dental treatment pay 80% of the cost of their treatment, up to a ceiling of £348; the government pays the remaining 20% and any additional sum above the £348 ceiling. Dentists are paid a fixed monthly sum for providing continuing care to all adult patients registered with them. The most recent fee for adults under 65 is 54 p (House of Commons Health Committee 2001). Dental treatment is provided on a fee-per-item basis. For non-exempt patients, the 80% of the cost of treatment is paid directly to the dentist by the patient. The remainder of any payment along with the cost of treatment for exempt patients is reimbursed through the Dental Practice Board on a monthly schedule.

Children receive free dental treatment and dentists are paid, in the majority, through a capitation system. When capitation was first introduced for children in 1990, there were entry payments for children prior to joining the capitation scheme to render them 'dentally fit'. Capitation payments were linked to the child's age but no weighting was given to children with higher than average disease levels. In 1996 the child item of service range was increased to include restorative care and since then entry payments have discontinued.

Patterns of registration and gross fees

After the introduction of the new contract in 1990, registration levels were 24.4 million. This declined steadily in the following years and has remained static at about 19.7 million for the last 3 years. Many patients are unaware that their registration 'lapses' after 15 months. As of May 1999, approximately 30 million patients were registered with 21 000 GDPs in the UK. Twenty-eight million people are registered (48% of the adult and 62% of child population) in England and Wales (Anon 1999), with over one-third of registered adults being exempt from patient charges. The latest figures can be obtained from the Dental Practice Board website (http://www.dpb.nhs.uk/dentaldata/index.html). The gross fees claimed by GDPs operating in the GDS in 1997/98 were £1344.4 million (Dental Practice Board 1990–1998). Of this, £985.4 million was claimed for adult treatment and £359 million for treatment of children. Gross fees for children's treatment (capitation and item of service) accounted for over a quarter of the gross fees claimed in England and Wales.

Regulation

As far back as 1960s there were concerns about the treatment emphasis of the GDS. By 1986 this concern had developed into suggestions that dentists were undertaking unnecessary dental treatments. The Schanschiff Report (1986) made 52 recommendations to improve the monitoring and regulation of the provision of care in the GDS. Following publication of the report, the Dental Reference Service, a unit within the Dental Practice Board, was strengthened. The Dental Reference Service employs a number of Dental Reference Officers, who ensure that any treatment carried out under NHS regulations is both necessary and provided to an appropriate standard. Patients who have had NHS treatment are randomly selected from every GDP and the quality of the practitioner's work assessed. The Dental Reference Service also has a role to play in prior approval: should an estimate for the cost of dental treatment exceed £200 the dentist is required to seek prior approval from the Dental Practice Board.

Training

Following graduation, any dentist wishing to work in the GDS is required to complete a 1-year vocational training course. This involves being assigned to a recognized training practice, and attending a day release course. The educational content of each course is not fixed nationally but topics that are generally covered include peer review, audit, practice management, and dental policy as well as clinical techniques. From 2001 dentists will have to undertake 250 hours of continuing professional education over a 5 year-period, 75 of which must be verifiable (see: http://www.gdc-uk.org/lifelong/LifeLongLearning.htm). In addition, new guidelines on peer review and clinical governance will require dentists to monitor the quality of their work and activities. (See the section 'Future issues facing dental care delivery' for a more detailed account of clinical governance.)

The Community Dental Service

The Community Dental Service (CDS) evolved out of the local authority priority dental service and did not become part of the NHS until 1974. The remit of the service was to treat school and pre-school children, and expectant and nursing mothers (Gelbier 1994). The school service accounted for 92% of its activities; the remaining 8% for expectant and nursing mothers was funded by the Department of Health (Gelbier 1998). The 1973 NHS Reorganization Act brought the service into the NHS and renamed it the Community Dental Service. The remit of the CDS was widened to include care for groups with special needs in addition to its remit in relation to children. By 1989 the role of the CDS had expanded again. It was now to act as a 'safety net' for people who could not access mainstream dental services, monitor trends in oral health of population through school screening and epidemiological surveys, provide health promotion, and act as a specialist referral service for the provision of general anaesthesia and orthodontics.

There are no registration arrangements such as exist for the GDS. Patients are identified through screening programmes, local epidemiological surveys, referrals, and local contracts. Once a patient has a relationship with a local dental clinic they tend to remain there for treatment. Children who are not 'special needs' are encouraged to register with local GDS dentists. Health authorities are responsible for making arrangements for CDSs with NHS Trusts. This can include Primary Care Trusts. They can also be administered

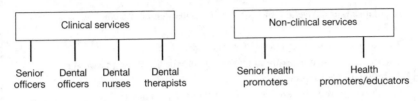

Fig. 19.4 Grade structure of staff employed in the CDS.

through directly managed units of the local health authority (Bradnock and Pine 1997).

Current remuneration arrangements

The CDS is a salaried service. Terms and conditions of service are negotiated through the joint negotiating forum for CDSs of the Whitely council. Remuneration is decided through the Dentists and Doctors Review Body. There are 1700 dentists employed in the CDS (Anon 1999), although the number of whole-time equivalents is less. Figure 19.4 illustrates the staff structure.

Regulation

Although a small service, the CDS is closely monitored through its contractual arrangements with the health authority and, if present, would be one of the responsibilities of the Consultant in Dental Public Health. A local health authority is not obliged to use the CDS.

Training requirements

As with the GDS, vocational training after qualification is a compulsory requirement for dentists employed in the CDS and staff are expected to undergo regular continuing professional education. For dentists wishing to obtain promotion within the CDS an appropriate postgraduate qualification is required (see Fig. 19.4).

The introduction of specialist registers in dentistry has implications for the CDS. It has been predicted that there will be 'specialists in community dental practice' who will provide care for young children, children and adults with mental, social, and physical handicaps, older people, and those who are housebound (Gelbier 1998). Such specialists will have recognition from the General Dental Council, and will require at least 3 years' formal training in recognized training posts.

The Personal Dental Services Scheme

The Personal Dental Services (PDS) pilot schemes were established in 1998 following changes in the Primary Care Act in the previous year that allowed

Box 19.2 Activities of specialists

1. Consultant advice to GDPs, GPs, community dental and community medical staff.
2. Acting as a point of referral for other specialities.
3. Undertaking complex treatment for patients who cannot receive care in a primary care setting.
4. Providing routine care for some special need patients.
5. Providing accident and emergency cover for dental infections and maxillo-facial trauma.
6. Providing dental care for inpatients in long-stay facilities.
7. Providing dental care for short-stay patients in facilities for the relief of pain and sepsis.

(Gelbier 1998)

alterations to the funding mechanisms. They were designed initially to examine differing methods of providing general dentistry. Details of the schemes can be found at the Department of Health website (http://www.doh.gov.uk/dental/schemes.htm). Importantly, the schemes remain pilots. The first-wave pilot arrangements were for 3 years, and are continuing. These projects represent local initiatives to solving local problems and often differ from each other. Some are examining changes to the remuneration system, adopting capitation-based mechanisms, while others involve differing skill-mix arrangements or the provision of selective treatments, for example orthodontics or dentures. Subsequent waves of PDS schemes have seen the conversion of CDS services to PDS, in part due to the creation of Primary Care Groups and Trusts which saw the funds for primary care health services move out from health authorities to the Primary Health Trusts.

The Hospital Dental Service

The Hospital Dental Service (HDS) employs approximately 2500 dentally qualified personnel (Anon 1999). It serves two functions: the provision of specialist dental care and the training of undergraduates and postgraduates. Box 19.2 describes the activities involved in specialist care.

There are strict contractual arrangements with the health authority for the provision of HDSs and it is estimated that the HDS provides about 7% of dental care in the UK (Bradnock and Pine 1997).

Current remuneration arrangements

Dentists operating with the HDS are salaried and salaries are set by the Dentists and Doctors Review Body. Consultants have parity with medical colleagues and similar staffing arrangements. Funds are in the majority derived through Part II funds. For those hospitals which have a teaching commitment, the additional funding required is paid for by the Service Increment for Teaching formula. Service Increment for Teaching money is provided nationally through the National Dental Service Increment for Teaching Purchasing Unit in Sheffield. Dental Schools and hospitals also receive money through research and development funds.

Regulation and training

The training of undergraduates and postgraduates is monitored by both the General Dental Council and the royal colleges, the latter acting as gatekeepers to consultant and specialist training. The General Dental Council makes visitations to accredit undergraduate training and lays down strict criteria for the training of consultants. In addition university education is monitored.

PRIVATE DENTAL CARE IN THE UK

While the majority of dental care is provided through the NHS, since the problems over the fee clawback in 1991/92 more dentists are believed to have moved over to private dental care. Current estimates suggest 24% of adult patients receive some or all of their dental treatment under private arrangements (British Dental Association 1998). Factors suggested as influencing this increase include: restricted availability of NHS treatment and a perception that private care is higher quality than NHS dental care (Blackburn 1999)

Structure

There are three ways in which people obtain private dental care from a dentist in the UK:

- Self-pay; that is, they pay for dental care out of their own pocket.
- Capitation arrangements.
- Dental insurance arrangements.

Self-pay private care

Dentists operating under self pay may charge any fee they choose, although a suggested tariff of fees is produced by the British Dental Association. The costs are usually based on a fixed charge per time unit plus any associated laboratory expenses. The majority of non-NHS care is provided through these arrangements, and in many cases in combination with NHS care.

Capitation plans

Capitation plans provide a level of care over a specified period for a specified sum of money. The patients' oral health is assessed and any treatment is provided prior to enrolling on the capitation scheme. The dentist decides at what level the patient will enter the plan and the cost of the plan will be set accordingly. Someone with a low disease history will pay a smaller sum than someone with high disease levels. The basis for this arrangement centres on the idea that the best predictor of future disease is past disease. Under capitation, the dentist has the incentive of encouraging greater preventative habits in their patients, thus reducing the need for restorative care.

Dental insurance arrangements

Indemnity insurance

The insurer underwrites the plan. The level of dental health is not known prior to the agreement. Patients are free to choose their dentist and type of treatment. The insurance covers the patient's treatment needs, which may include extensive restorative care. Premiums are thus higher than capitation. There is no preventive incentive. The patient pays the dentist directly for dental treatment and is then reimbursed by the insurance company making a claim.

Cash plan insurance

Cash plans provide cash benefits towards primary care. Some plans specialize in providing benefits for dental treatment only, but the majority provide for a range of primary care services that would include dental care. The plan is usually renewed annually and provides cash up to a maximum level to cover dental treatment.

Dental payment plans

A dental payment plan typically take place within individual practices. It is not an insurance scheme, since patients pay the full cost of treatment. It does, however, allow the patient to spread the cost of treatment over time. It is particularly useful for expensive courses of treatment such as orthodontic fixed appliance therapy or complex crown and bridge work.

Corporate bodies

Besides individual dentists, there are a limited number of 'companies' that can provide dental services. These companies have to meet one additional requirement that differentiates them from other companies: the majority of directors have to be dentally qualified. At present there are 27 corporate bodies that were 'grandfathered' before the 1952 Dentists Act prevented the creation of additional corporates. Few currently have more than five dental practices and growth on any scale is limited to four corporates (Blackburn 1999). Recently, there has been a great interest in corporate bodies as these are the only way a company (aside from a dentist) can deliver dental care. Economies of scale and a quality brand name are the main reason for companies to work to establish dental practices (Blackburn 1999).

Regulation

The practice of private dentistry is not subject to the same controls that operate in the NHS. Indeed, for any transaction that does not involve a third party, if the patient cannot get satisfaction following a complaint to the practitioner, the only recourse is a court of law or the General Dental Council. Where a third party is involved, for example Denplan (http://www.denplan.co.uk/), more stringent controls are in place.

PROFESSIONS COMPLEMENTARY TO DENTISTRY (PCDS)

For many years, doctors have been used to working with a considerable number of allied professions for example, medical physicists, speech therapists, and physiotherapists. Doctors are used to diagnosing a problem and then referring for specific items of treatment. In recent years these professions have developed considerable expertise and often undertake parts of the diagnosis for themselves.

In dentistry the development of allied professions has been much slower, and dentists have retained almost all of the operative work for themselves. However, dentists are expensive to train and employ and a considerable proportion of their tasks are fairly routine and of low skill level. Hygienists were readily accepted by the profession but other groups have been less readily welcomed.

Types of PCDs

Within the UK these are:
- dental nurses;
- dental hygienists;
- dental therapists;
- dental technicians.

Each of these is governed by legislation that is also of relevance to the dentist regarding their permitted clinical functions. Dental hygienists and dental therapists are known as operating dental auxiliaries as they are presently the only categories who are allowed to treat patients. The range of treatments that they are permitted to provide is specified in regulations which are amended in the light of clinical advancement. For example, dental hygienists were not initially permitted to give any form of local anaesthesia but are now permitted to give infiltration anaesthesia under the direct personal supervision of a dentist. These two groups of staff may only work to the prescription of a dentist and as such are not permitted to diagnose or prescribe treatment themselves.

Dental hygienists may work in all areas of dental practice but dental therapists are limited to hospital, community, or personal dental services.

The duties of these groups are described in a consultation paper (General Dental Council 1998):

Dental hygienists may clean, scale and polish teeth and apply prophylactic materials to the teeth to the written prescription of a registered dentist, as well as providing dental health education. They are also permitted to administer local infiltration analgesia under the direct personal supervision of a registered dentist.

Dental therapists are permitted to extract deciduous teeth, undertake simple dental fillings, clean and polish teeth, scale teeth and apply prophylactic materials to the teeth. They are also permitted to administer local infiltration analgesia. Dental therapists work to the written prescription of a registered dentist but, currently, only within the hospital and community dental services.

Practitioners in both groups are required to be enrolled with the General Dental Council.

The Nuffield Foundation (1993), in its enquiry on this subject, described three objectives of a comprehensive service:

- promoting oral health of both individuals and communities by information, advice, practical help, and liaison with general health care;
- providing readily available treatment for those who do not yet have good oral health;
- maintaining the good health of those who enjoy it.

Purpose

This describes the duties of these PCDs, but what is their purpose? Why are they needed in addition to dentists? The Nuffield Report said that it was convinced that a more effective service might be provided within cash limits if greater numbers of these groups of staff were employed. Within British dentistry the concept of the need for a team approach to the provision of dental care is becoming more accepted as being desirable. In essence this sees the need to divide tasks between different members of the team, depending upon their areas of skill and expertise. At its best, the dentist would undertake the examination, diagnosis, and prescription of the care required for the patient and then delegate various duties to the team members. The dentist would then be able to concentrate on those tasks for which only dentists are qualified.

DISCUSSION POINTS

What benefits can you see for the patient and the dentist in the development of team dentistry? You should look at the objectives of a health service listed above.

The Nuffield Report also recommended the registration of dental nurses and the creation of other groups of PCDs, namely dental technicians who can make full dentures, and orthodontic auxiliaries.

The development of PCDs has been severely restricted by the numbers in training and the opportunities that are available. Until these factors are changed it is unlikely that there will be much development in this area.

FUTURE ISSUES FACING DENTAL CARE DELIVERY

The vision for dentistry proposed by the government was outlined in *Modernising NHS dentistry – implementing the plan* (Department of Health 2000). The key issues identified were ensuring access to care, improving the quality of care, and reducing inequalities in oral health. These issues are synonymous with the themes for the reform of the NHS in general.

To address access issues, the government has invested in the infrastructure necessary for care by building dental access centres. Unlike conventional dental practices, patients will not need to register to obtain care. Whether this will have a major impact remains to be seen. A further question surrounds the workforce: current working practices limit the scope for change and a review of personnel requirements is underway. Issues that will need to be considered include the numbers, types, and working arrangements of all grades of oral health care workers to ensure that the care system operates efficiently.

The quality agenda is being addressed through the implementation of clinical governance. From 2001, clinical governance is part of the terms and conditions of service for GDPs working in the GDS. Clinical governance has a number of arms but can be described as ensuring that a patient receives optimal care. The government published the consultation document, *Supporting doctors, protecting patient* (Department of Health 1998), and invited views on its proposals to radically reform the existing arrangements for preventing, recognizing, and dealing with the poor clinical performance. Following consultation, the government has created a number of bodies that will be responsible for ensuring the quality of care is appropriate. These bodies include the National Institute for Clinical Excellence (NICE), the Commission for Health Improvement (CHI), and the National Care Standards Commission.

How to reduce inequalities, and in particular what the role of oral health care services is, continues to be a key issue. A number of initiatives based loosely on the primary health care approach are underway, working through the Health Action Zones (http://www.haznet.org.uk/). There is also continued discussion on the fluoridation of water supplies.

A further question concerns both the number and type of personnel required to provide oral health care. With the decline in disease the arguments for a different skill-mixed workforce based on increased numbers of PCDs becomes stronger. This has large implications for training and working arrangements. But perhaps the biggest question centres on the extent to which government should pay for oral health care. Already the Dutch and Swedish governments have decided that the state should reduce its commitment to providing adult dental care. With other health priorities and limits to the resources available, the arguments to support state provision of dental care will need to be made.

CONCLUSION

There are a number of ways in which the provision of care can be organized. All systems have a basic structure: an initial method of allocating resources, their subsequent distribution, monitoring arrangements, and educational arrangements. Resources can be allocated by an individual to pay for care, or be pooled through the collection of premiums or taxes. No country leaves dental care entirely up to the individual although differing priority groups exist.

Methods for paying dental care workers are limited to four main mechanisms: fee-per-item, capitation, salaried, or on a sessional basis. Irrespective of the method of payment supporting structures are required. These include the information systems, probity mechanisms, and training system.

In the UK, the major provider of care is the GDS. The system is funded through taxation although cost sharing for non-exempt groups exists. Dentists are paid in the majority on a fee-per-item arrangement as independent contractors. Other providers of care include the CDS and HDS, the former providing care to priority groups and undertaking screening and epidemiological activities. The latter service provides specialist care as well as being responsible for training.

REFERENCES

Anon (1999). BDA gives evidence on regulation of private care. *British Dental Association News,* **12** (3).

Batchelor, P. and Sterling, D. (1998). *UK dental services.* Paper presented at the annual scientific conference of the British Association for the Study of Community Dentistry, pp. 1–46.

Bearne, A. (1998). Part-time or private? *British Dental Association News,* **11** (10), pp. 1–32

Blackburn, P. (1999) *UK Dental Care.* Laing and Buisson

Bloomfield Report (1992). *Fundamental review of dental remuneration.* London, HMSO.

Bradnock, G. and Pine, C. (1997) Delivery of oral health care and implications for future planning: in the UK. In *Community oral health* (ed. C. Pine), pp. 267–306. Oxford, Wright.

Dental Practice Board (1990–98). *Gross fees: GDS annual statistics.* Bournemouth, Dental Practice Board.

Department of Health (1998) *Supporting doctors, protecting patients. A consultation paper on preventing, recognising and dealing with poor clinical performance of doctors in the NHS in England.* London, Stationery Office.

Department of Health (2000) *Modernising Dentistry: Implementing the NHS plan.* London, Stationery Office.

Gelbier, S. (1994). Where have we come from? In *Introduction to dental public health* (ed. M. Downer, S. Gelbier, and D. Gibbons), pp. 11–29. London, FDI World Dental Press.

Gelbier, S (1998). The present and future role of the Community Dental Service. *Community Dental Health,* **15** (Suppl. 1), 306–11.

General Dental Council (1998). *Professionals complementary to dentistry.* Consultation paper. London.

House of Commons Health Committee (1993). *Fourth report on dental services 1993.* London, HMSO.

House of Commons Health Committee (2001). *First report on access to NHS dentistry 2001.* http://www.publications.parliament.uk/pa/cm200001/cmselect/cmhealth/247.htm

National Health Service Executive (1997). *Personal dental services pilots.* London, HMSO.

Nuffield Foundation (1993). *Education and training of personnel auxiliary to dentistry.* London, Nuffield Foundation.

Schanschiff Report (1986). *Report of the Committee of Inquiry into Unnecessary Dental Treatment.* Department of Health and Social Security. London, HMSO.

Todd, J. and Lader, D. (1991) *Adult Dental Health 1988.* United Kingdom OPCS, London HMSO.

20 The European Union and dentistry

CONTENTS

By the end of this chapter you should be able to:

- Understand the basic structure of the European Union.
- Describe the relevance of the European Union to the practice of dentistry.

This chapter links with:
- Introduction to the principles of dental health (Chapter 1).
- Organization of health care (Chapter 10).

INTRODUCTION

As the UK is part of the European Union it is important to understand the effect this has on the practice of dentistry within the UK. This chapter briefly reviews the European Union legislation as it relates to dentistry, and describes common features found in European states with regard to the practice of dentistry.

BASIC LEGISLATION AND ORGANIZATIONS

The European Union consists of 15 member states with over 370 million citizens.

The European Commission

The body responsible for developing and proposing European Union policy and legislation which is then discussed, adopted, and amended by the Council of Ministers. The Commission then implements the decision and is, therefore, the civil service of the European Union. There are 20 commissioners (two each from Germany, Spain, France, Italy and the UK and one from each of the other states). The Commission is divided into 24 Directorates-General and is staffed by career officials. Matters relevant to dentists and dental services cross directorate boundaries.

The Council

The Council is the European Union's decision-maker, adopting or amending the Commission's proposals. The term 'council' covers a variety of organizations including the Council of Ministers but also the specialist councils and committees of permanent representatives of the member states in Brussels.

The European Parliament

This is a directly elected body of 626 members from all member states. Although its power has increased with the Single European Act, its role remains largely advisory given the roles of the Commission and the Council. The parliament can propose amendments but a unanimous vote in Council remains the final voice. The parliament has the power, with a two-thirds majority, to dismiss the Council. It also has some input into the budgetary process and can set up commissions of inquiry.

The Court of Justice

This is made up of 15 independent judges, with at least one from each member state. It has two roles: to ensure that any actions of national governments or institutions that conflict with European Union treaties are stopped and to pass judgement on cases referred by national courts.

The Economic and Social Committee

Based in Brussels, this is a consultative body of 222 members representing employers, trade unions, and other interested bodies such as farmers and consumers. The Commission is required to take note of its opinion on proposals relating to economic and social matters.

TYPES OF EUROPEAN LEGISLATION

Whitehouse *et al.* (2000) report the types of legislation available in Europe:
- *Regulations*: apply to all member states and do not have to be approved by the national government.
- *Directives*: are compulsory but the member states have to translate them into national legislation.
- *Decisions*: only binding on the body or individual to which they are addressed
- *Recommendations and Opinions*: these are not binding and state the view of the issuing body.

DENTISTRY AND THE EUROPEAN UNION

Article 129 of the Treaty of Rome requires the European Union:
- To contribute towards ensuring a high level of human health protection.
- To direct action towards the prevention of diseases, particularly, of the major health scourges, including drug dependence, by promoting research into their causes and transmission as well as health information and education.

One area in which the European Union works is by funding collaborative research between member states, for which major research schemes are available. It is not yet clear what the European Union's role will be in public health although there are developments in this area.

FREEDOM OF MOVEMENT

In 1969, the principle of freedom of movement was established and aimed to 'abolish any discrimination based on nationality between workers of the Member States as regards employment, remuneration and other conditions of work and employment'.

This means that every worker who is a citizen of a member state has the right to:
- Accept offers of employment in any European Union country.
- Move freely within the European Union for the purposes of employment.
- Be employed in a country in accordance with the provisions governing the employment of nationals of that country.
- Remain in the country after the employment ceases (Whitehouse *et al.* 2000).

The freedom of movement has applied to dentists since 1980, if their education has met the requirements of the Dental Directives.

THE DENTAL DIRECTIVES

The European Union Dental Directives (78/686 and 687 EEC) mean that any national of a member state who holds one of the recognized qualifications of dentistry may practise dentistry in any other member state. Under the European Economic Area agreement Norway, Iceland, and Liechtenstein are also included.

The Dental Directives outline that the course of training must be a minimum of 5 years in a university or university equivalent. The course must include theoretical and practical work and a list of the subjects that should be covered. Member states are not allowed to place restrictions on incoming dentists; for example, language requirements. However, incoming dentists may be expected to comply with any restrictions placed on local dentists.

To practice in another country dentists must register with the competent authority in the country in which they work; in the UK this is the General Dental Council. Each country has an information body that will provide details of the registration procedure. A full list of these is given in (Whitehouse *et al.* 2000).

SPECIFIC REQUIREMENTS RELATING TO REGISTRATION

- *Good character and good repute: a* certificate must be provided indicating that the dentist is of good standing in his/her own state. The new state may request an extract from the 'judicial record' or an equivalent document.

- *Serious professional misconduct and criminal penalties*: all information must be forwarded to the new state.
- *Physical and mental health*: some states require evidence of satisfactory health.
- *Duration of the authorizing procedure:* must be completed within 3 months of application. This period may be altered if there are any doubts about any of the above matters.
- *Alternative to taking an oath*: if an oath or solemn declaration is required in order to practice, an alternative must be offered if the former is inappropriate for the individual.

SPECIALIZATION IN EUROPE

To be accepted as a speciality, a discipline must be recognized in two or more member states. Currently, only two specialities meet this criteria, orthodontics and oral surgery. Training as a specialist must be on a full-time course of 3 years' duration in a university or otherwise approved establishment. The trainee must be individually supervised.

The criteria for both postgraduate and undergraduate study are the minimum training requirements. A member state may impose additional criteria for qualifications acquired within its territory. It must not impose additional requirements on people gaining qualifications in other member states.

DENTAL PRACTICE IN EUROPE

The practice of dentistry in each of the states of Europe is different but there are some common themes. In Europe, dental care is provided mainly by 'general' or 'liberal' practitioners. Only in Scandinavia and Ireland are there more than 20% of dentists working in areas other than general practice. Access to oral health care is still largely determined by the distribution of dentists. Some governments or other bodies offer financial assistance, but this is usually limited to a standard package of care. Dentists are paid on a fee-per-service basis.

All countries have dental nurses, although they are recognized by a variety of names. Dental technicians are recognized in all countries and hygienists in most. However, only a few countries recognize any other type of auxiliary.

RECENT DEVELOPMENTS

The reforms of health care in Europe are based on two main themes: decentralization of the management of public services and higher patient charges

(Holst *et al.* 2001). The degree to which any member state has autonomy over these moves is unclear. Challenges to the limitations that European Union member states place on care entitlements to their citizens have been challenged in the European Court of Justice (Watson 1998) in two cases. These cases arose from Luxembourg and sought the right for citizens of European Union member states to seek care in any of the member states. The first case covered optical services brought by Nicolas Decker, the second, an orthodontic case brought by Raymond Kohl. The court ruled that citizens of the European Union could seek care in any other member state. The implications of this case may be far-reaching as governments attempt to limit the care entitlement to their citizens.

CONCLUSION

The European Union offers opportunities for dentists in education, research, and practice. European Union legislation is an influencing factor on the practice of dentistry and this is likely to become of greater importance as member states move closer together.

REFERENCES

Holst, D., Sheiham, A., and Petersen, P. E. (2001). Oral health care services in Europe. Some recent changes and a public health perspective. *Zeitschrift für Gesundheitswiss,* **9**, 112–21.

Watson, R. (1998). Court rules that patients can seek treatment in any EU country. *British Medical Journal,* **316**, 1407.

Whitehouse, N. H. and Treasure, E. T. (1998). Dentistry and the National Health Service in the context of Europe. *British Dental Journal,* **185** (1), 30–2.

Whitehouse, N. M., Anderson, R., Treasure, E. T. *et al* (2000) *Dental Liasion Committee in the European Union: A practical guide to the oral health systems and current practice of dentistry in the eighteen different countries.* Cardiff, European Union Manual of Dental Practice.

FURTHER READING

Anderson, R., Treasure, E. T., Whitehouse, N. H., *et al.* (1998). Oral health systems in Europe. Part I: Finance and entitlement to care. *Community Dental Health,* **15** (3), 145–9.

Anderson, R., Treasure, E. T., Whitehouse, N. H., *et al.* (1998). Oral health systems in Europe. Part II: The dental workforce. *Community Dental Health,* **15** (4), 243–7.

21 Planning dental services

CONTENTS

INTRODUCTION

Planning is an integral part of dental care provision that can operate at many different levels. At a national level, government NHS policy impacts upon dental services in different ways. For example, a national payment system for General Dental Service patient charges is set by government. At a health authority level, planners make decisions over the types and range of services offered by the local hospital and community dental services. Within a dental practice, dental practitioners and their team members may develop a range of practice policies aimed at improving the services provided. Finally, every day clinicians develop treatment plans for individual patient care based upon their oral health needs. All these activities are planning in action.

This chapter will examine the basic principles of planning, and review the different steps in the planning process. Particular emphasis will be placed upon the assessment of need and the range of measures of oral health that can be used. In addition, the concept of quality of dental care and clinical governance will be explored.

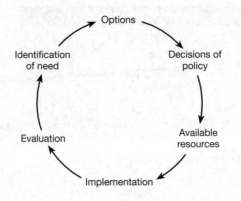

Fig. 21.1 Rational planning model. (Reproduced from McCarthy 1982 with permission from the King's Fund. See Permissions.)

PRINCIPLES OF PLANNING

At the most basic level, planning aims to guide choices so that decisions are made in the best manner to reach the desired outcomes. Planning provides a guide and structure to the process of decision-making to maximize results within the limited resources available. Is planning really necessary when there are so many other demands on practitioners' time?

Planning can be justified for the following reasons:

- It provides an opportunity to be proactive in decision-making rather than constantly reacting to pressures and demands.
- It enables priorities to be set.
- It identifies where resources can be directed to have the greatest impact.

Various planning models have been proposed to act as a guide to the different steps in the planning process. The rational planning model (see Fig. 21.1) provides a basic guide to the process (McCarthy 1982), and involves the following steps:

1. Assessment of need: identification of the oral health problems and concerns of the population.
2. Identifying priorities: agreeing the target areas for action.
3. Developing aims and objectives: aim is the overall goal to be achieved, whereas the objectives are the steps needed to reach the aim.
4. Assessing resources: identifying the range of resources available to facilitate implementation of the plan; for example, personnel, materials, and equipment.
5. Implementation: turning the plans into action.
6. Evaluation: measuring the changes resulting from the plan.

In reality planning is never straightforward. Information is often limited, there are pressures to focus on particular issues, and options may be restricted by a lack of resources. Often the potential for change is limited. A

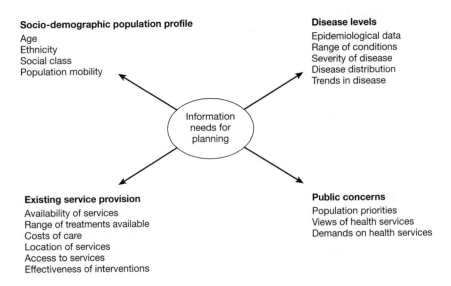

Socio-demographic population profile
Age
Ethnicity
Social class
Population mobility

Disease levels
Epidemiological data
Range of conditions
Severity of disease
Disease distribution
Trends in disease

Information
needs for
planning

Existing service provision
Availability of services
Range of treatments available
Costs of care
Location of services
Access to services
Effectiveness of interventions

Public concerns
Population priorities
Views of health services
Demands on health services

Fig. 21.2 Basic information used in health planning.

rational plan is therefore uncommon. Instead an incremental approach to planning is how decisions are made. This involves making small decisions based upon circumstances rather than grand plans for the future (McCarthy 1982).

In dentistry different models of, or approaches to, planning apply across the different service sectors. Within the Community and Hospital Dental Services the rational planning model is used to a certain extent. In the General Dental Service the dental practitioners need to plan how best to provide a good level of dental care, and make a reasonable income. Rational planning is therefore essential. You have to know what the dental problems are in the area where you practice, the attitudes, beliefs, and economic factors affecting demand, and the approaches your practice will adopt to best cope with the problems.

INFORMATION REQUIREMENTS FOR PLANNING

Access to a range of types of information is required (see Fig. 21.2) before informed planning decisions can be made.

DISCUSSION POINTS

Before setting up a new dental practice what types of information would a general dental practitioner require?

Where would this information be available?

ORAL HEALTH NEEDS ASSESSMENT

Defining and assessing need is a critical element of the planning process, and many definitions of need have been proposed. A very useful definition is:

> A need for medical care exists when an individual has an illness or disability for which there is an effective and acceptable treatment or cure. (Matthew 1972)

Bradshaw's (1972) taxonomy of need also provides a definition of the differing concepts of need. In this he defines 'normative need' as that which the professional or expert defines as need in a given situation. 'Felt need' or want is a lay person's own assessment of his or her needs. 'Expressed need' or demand is felt need translated into action, either by use of services or request for information. 'Comparative need' is assessed by comparing the health needs of similar groups of people.

DISCUSSION POINTS

Provide an oral health example of Bradshaw's concept of need for:
- Normative need
- Felt need
- Expressed need
- Comparative need

Traditionally oral health services have been planned on the basis of information collected in normative assessments of need. Professionally determined biomedical measures of disease such as DMF/dmf and Community Periodontal Index of treatment need (CPITN) indices have been extensively used to determine oral health needs. (Chapter 5 outlines in detail the epidemiological indices used in oral health measurement.)

Assessing oral health needs solely based upon normative measures has, however, certain fundamental shortcomings:

1. Normative assessments of need are not objective but rather based upon a wide range of factors with considerable inter- and intra-examiner variability.
2. Professional measures of oral diseases do not provide any information on the impact of disease on an individual's quality of life.
3. Ethically it is now considered unacceptable that need should be determined solely based upon professional judgements. With greater professional accountability and consumerism, health care decisions are now required to be more publicly agreed through a degree of consensus.
4. Normative needs have been criticized for their paradoxical approach. Ethically it is unacceptable to assess need and recommend treatment

when health care resources are not always available to meet this demand.

SOCIODENTAL MEASURES OF ORAL HEALTH

Recognition of the limitations of professionally defined need have led to the development of broader measures of health need based upon the concepts of impairment, disability, and handicap (Locker 1988; WHO 1980). These sociodental measures of oral health encompass social, functional, and other quality of life indicators.

DISCUSSION POINTS

Outline the range of ways in which oral diseases may have an impact on an individual's quality of life.

Sociodental measures are defined by Locker (1989) as 'measures of the extent to which dental and oral disorders disrupt normal social role functioning and bring about major changes in behaviour such as an inability to work or attend school, or undertake parental or household duties'. A range of sociodental measures have now been developed and tested. Table 21.1 lists several well known ones.

When indicators of social and psychological impact have been compared with clinical variables, a generally weak association has been found (Sheiham and Spencer 1997). To fully assess oral health needs therefore requires clinical measures as well as a selection of social and psychological indicators.

QUALITY OF DENTAL CARE AND CLINICAL GOVERNANCE

One of the key elements in planning dental services is to ensure that the quality of care provided is of the highest quality. In health services throughout the world efforts are being employed to examine the quality of services and identify opportunities for improvement. In the UK clinical governance is a key government priority for the development of the NHS (Department of Health 1997). Clinical governance can be defined as an ongoing programme aimed at changing the culture of the whole NHS and improving the quality of its services. Key components of clinical governance include:
- Clear lines of responsibility for the quality of clinical care.
- A comprehensive programme of activity which improves quality.
- Clear policies for managing risk.
- Procedures for all health care professionals to identify and remedy poor performance.

Table 21.1 Some well known sociodental measures

Sociodental measure	Authors	Impacts
Social Impacts of Dental Disease (SIDD)	Cushing et al. 1986	*Functional*: e.g. eating *Social Interaction*: e.g. communication *Comfort and well-being*: e.g. pain and discomfort *Self image*: e.g. aesthetics
Dental Impact Profile (DIP)	Strauss 1988	*Eating*: e.g. chewing and biting; food choice *Health/well-being*: e.g. feeling comfortable; appetite *Social Relations*: e.g. facial appearance; speech and breath; confidence around others *Romance*: e.g. social life; having sex appeal; kissing
Geriatric Oral Health Index of Assessment (GOHAI)	Atchison and Dolan 1990	*Eating* limit food due to dental problems; trouble biting and chewing *Pain*: used medication; sensitive to temperature *Social dimension*: nervous due to teeth; uncomfortable eating with people; prevented from speaking; worried about teeth; limited contacts with people
Oral Health Impact Profile (OHIP)	Slade and Spencer 1994	*Functional limitation*: e.g. difficulty chewing *Physical pain*: toothache *Psychological discomfort*: self conscious about mouth *Physical disability*: avoiding certain foods *Social disability*: avoided going out due to dental problems *Handicap*: financial loss
Dental Impacts on Daily Living (DIDL)	Leao and Sheiham 1995	*Appearance*: satisfaction with look of teeth *Comfort*: bad breath *Pain*: toothache *Performance*: ability to work/study *Eating restriction*: ability to chew and bite foods

Box 21.1 Local oral health planning example

The following is based on a actual example in an English town and provides a 'real life' situation in which planning decisions and processes were implemented.
Elements of the plan have been altered to make points for illustration.

Needs assessment
The routine epidemiological survey of 5-year-old children was used to map the disease level across the town.

Description of population
The town had a population of around 100 000 people. Due to the closure of various industries in previous years, unemployment was above the national average.
An area of the town was inhabited almost entirely by people of Bangladeshi origin. The majority of the adults in this area were first generation and many of the women did not speak any English. This community was within easy walking distance of the town centre, supermarket, and general dental practitioners. However, the religion of this community was Islam and although the mothers took the children to school they were not permitted to leave the house for other reasons.
There was a large housing estate on the periphery of the town where unemployment was very high, and it was recognized as one of the most deprived areas within the region. There were also some areas of commuter-belt housing which were relatively advantaged.
The entire population received fluoridated water.

Resource assessment
The distribution of general dental practitioners was mapped on top of the disease levels, as was the current deployment of Community Dental Service staff. At the start of the process there were no problems for adults in accessing general dental practitioners as all were accepting new adult patients.

Defining the problems
There was a very high level of decay, untreated, among the children of Bangladeshi origin. Uptake of services in this community was low. There was a similar but less severe problem in the deprived housing estate. However, the previous year's survey had shown this estate to have very high disease levels in 12-year-old children. The general practitioner and the community dentist were both well accepted by the population but were both working to capacity.
The CDS was in a time of financial restriction with cuts being planned every year. Any plan had to be, at best, resource neutral. Resources available to the Community Dental Service were the three dentists working in the town and two dentists and one therapist working outside of the town. There were two mobile dental units.

> **DISCUSSION POINTS**
>
> Given the data above, what actions might be possible in order to achieve some health improvements and to solve some of the problems? Consider preventive strategies and alterations to treatment provision that might assist.
>
> What political, cultural, and social problems might you encounter?

The recently published Dental Strategy for England has outlined ways forward for clinical governance in dentistry (Department of Health 2000). Governments, funding organizations, and the public expect, and increasingly demand, reassurance that quality issues are being reviewed and maintained within health services. Quality of care is and will remain a central issue for all health professionals. However, what do we mean by 'quality', and in what ways can this be examined and improved upon?

Definitions of quality

Before considering methods of improving the quality of a service, it is fundamentally important to have an agreed definition of quality.

> **DISCUSSION POINTS**
>
> Consider a transport system that is familiar to you. Perhaps a metro system, bus service, or rail network. What would be the features of a high-quality transport system?
>
> Consider this from three different perspectives:
> - a passenger's viewpoint;
> - an employee of the transport system, e.g. train driver, ticket inspector;
> - a director of the management board.
>
> Generate a list of features of quality from each of these perspectives and then compare and contrast your findings.
>
> Finally, check to see if your list of quality features applies to how the quality of health services would be described. Apart from some differences in terminology, for example, patients rather than passengers, do many of the issues apply to any service?

Defining quality of health care involves a range of different areas and is not an easy task. When clinicians are asked to propose a definition of quality they tend to concentrate very much on the technical and scientific elements of treatment. These, of course, reflect the nature and focus of professional training and expertise. However, from a public health perspective quality of dental care encompasses much more than the cavosurface angle in a cavity preparation, or the precision of a marginal ridge in an amalgam restoration. Defining quality of care is not the sole prerogative of clinicians; users of services and health services managers and planners also have an important contribution to make. Maxwell (1984) has proposed a definition of quality which has been widely accepted as reflecting the breadth and complexity of this topic.

The definition has the following components:

1. *Effectiveness*: that services achieve their intended benefit. For example, that orthodontic treatment produces a long-term, sustained improvement in malocclusion.
2. *Access*: that the services are easily available to users in terms of time, cost, distance, and ethos; for example, ensuring that different users of services such as disabled people can utilize dental care.
3. *Socially acceptable*: that services are provided to satisfy the reasonable expectations of users, providers and the community; for example, in areas where English is not the first language of many people, services should recognize this and provide information and resources in an appropriate language and format.
4. *Efficiency and economy*: that the services achieve maximum benefit for minimum cost; for example, by limiting wasteful use of materials and equipment.
5. *Relevance to need*: that the service is what the users actually need; for example, that dental services provided reflect the needs of local population, such as prosthetic care for an area with a large number of older people.
6. *Equity*: that services will be fairly directed to those in need; for example, dental services should be available to all groups in society not just those with private health insurance.

Another popular definition of quality was proposed by the Royal College of General Practitioners (1985) when they reviewed what would be the core features of a high-quality service provided by a general medical practitioner. This definition has more of a clinical focus and encompasses the following features:

1. *Interpersonal skills*: the ability to communicate effectively with users and colleagues is an essential component of clinical practice.
2. *Clinical competence*: the ability to perform core clinical tasks to a sufficient standard to ensure the effective and safe delivery of appropriate care.
3. *Professional values*: this recognizes the importance of ethical and professional principles relevant to the delivery of health care. These include respect for clients' rights and autonomy, justice, beneficence, confidentiality, and privacy.
4. *Access*: the ability of clients to utilize and benefit from care is a fundamental requirement.

Finally, Donabedian (1974) describes quality of health care as having three inter-related elements: structure, process, and outcome.

- *Structure* refers to the physical elements of care such as the facilities, equipment, and premises.
- *Process* involves all the various ways in which the system deals with people using the service. This includes the clinical techniques employed, the administrative and management systems, and the appointments procedures.
- *Outcome* refers to the consequences of contact with the service; in other words, what has changed as a result of using the service. For example, has the toothache stopped?

Whichever definition of quality is used, it is very important that it encompasses the range of potential concerns of clinicians, service users, and health service managers.

Implementing quality within dental services

Improving the quality of dental care is a challenging and time-consuming process. It requires clinicians to critically appraise their own performances and to share their expertise and knowledge with colleagues. Continuing professional development, peer review, and clinical audit are all elements of clinical governance (Department of Health 2000).

The audit cycle provides a useful structure to follow when considering the best means of improving service performance. Figure 21.3 provides a diagrammatic outline of the different steps in the audit cycle.

When establishing a quality team it is essential that ground rules are agreed to promote trust, understanding, and respect. Issues such as confidentiality need to be addressed and procedures agreed. Initially it is best to focus on relatively straightforward areas for review. Once confidence and expertise are developed more challenging areas of practice can be tackled.

Setting and agreeing standards of care is a critical step in the audit process. This can be a very time-consuming and difficult task, especially reaching a consensus view. Gaining access to the scientific literature and existing published professional guidelines can facilitate the task of setting clear, precise, and up-to-date standards of care.

Probably the most problematic step in the audit cycle is developing and implementing the system of monitoring practice against agreed standards of care. Set criteria need to be developed to measure practice performance once the quality standards are agreed. These criteria must be objective, reliable, and rigorous. When practice is compared with the set standards and found to be inadequate, appropriate action needs to be taken. In most cases this may involve accessing training and support, or changing certain types of equipment or materials used.

Reviewing the value of the quality system is essential in ensuring that it provides real benefits to all members of the team, and most importantly, to the service that is delivered to practice users. A variety of materials have

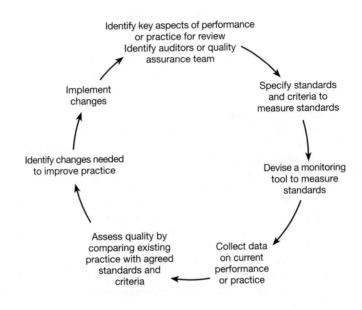

Fig. 21.3 Quality assurance cycle. (Reproduced with permission from Ewles and Simnett 1999. See Permissions.)

been designed to help dentists review and improve quality of care (Department of Health 2001; Faculty of Dental Surgery 1991; Faculty of General Dental Practitioners 1996).

CONCLUSION

Within a constantly changing world, planning is an essential activity to ensure that dental care responds and develops appropriately to the new challenges presented. Assessing need is at the core of planning. It is critical that any needs assessment encompasses a broad definition of need. Sociodental measures of oral health provide a useful means of assessing the impact of oral diseases on individuals and communities. Internationally, health services are striving to improve the quality of care provided. Within dentistry clinical governance mechanisms are now being introduced which seek to review and implement improvements in the standards and quality of dental care. Again it is important that any efforts to improve quality of care encompass a broad and balanced definition of quality which includes the perspectives of clinicians, service users, and health service managers.

REFERENCES

Atchison, K. and Dolan, T. (1990). Development of the geriatric oral health assessment index. *Journal of Dental Education*, **54**, 680–7.

Bradshaw, J. (1972). A taxonomy of social need. In *Problems and progress in medical care* (ed. G. McLachlan), pp. 69–82. Oxford, Oxford University Press.

Cushing, A., Sheiham, A., and Maizels, J. (1986). Developing socio-dental indicators – the social impact of dental disease. *Community Dental Health*, **3**, 3–17.

Department of Health (1997). *The new NHS: modern, dependable*. London, The Stationery Office.

Department of Health (2000). *Modernising NHS dentistry – implementing the NHS plan*. London, Department of Health.

Department of Health (2001). *Clinical audit and peer review in the GDS*. London, Department of Health.

Donabedian, A. (1974). *Aspects of medical care administration: specifying requirements for health care*. Cambridge, Mass, Harvard University Press.

Ewles, L. and Simnett, I (1992) *Promoting Health: a practical guide*. London, Scutari Press.

Faculty of Dental Surgery (1991). *Clinical standards in general dental practice: self assessment manual and standards*. London, Faculty of Dental Surgery.

Faculty of General Dental Practitioners (1996). *An anatomy of general dental practice: the structure and process*. London, Faculty of General Dental Practitioners.

Leao, A. and Sheiham, A. (1995). Relation between clinical dental status and subjective impacts on daily living. *Journal of Dental Research*, **74**, 1408–13.

Locker, D. (1988). Measuring oral health: a conceptual framework. *Community Dental Health*, **5**, 3–18.

Locker, D. (1989). *An introduction to behavioural science and dentistry*. London, Routledge.

McCarthy, M. (1982). *Epidemiology and policies for health planning*. London, King Edward's Hospital Fund for London.

Matthew, G. (1971). Measuring need and evaluating services. In *Portfolio for health* (ed. G. McLachlan), pp. 83–99. Oxford, Oxford University Press.

Maxwell, R. (1984). Quality assessment in health. *British Medical Journal*, **288**, 1470–72.

Royal College of General Practitioners (1985). *What sort of doctor?* Report from general practice No 23. London, Royal College of General Practitioners.

Sheiham, A. and Spencer, J. (1997). Health needs assessment. In *Community oral health* (ed. C. Pine), pp. 39–54. Oxford, Wright.

Slade, G. and Spencer, J. (1994). Development and evaluation of the Oral Health Impact Profile. *Community Dental Health*, **11**, 3–11.

Strauss, R. (1988). The patient with cancer: social and clinical perspectives for the dentist. *Special Care Dentistry*, **8**, 129–34.

WHO (World Health Organization) (1980). *International classification of impairments, disabilities and handicaps*. Geneva, WHO.

FURTHER READING

Coast, J., Donovan, J., and Frankel, S. (1996). *Priority setting: the health care debate*. Chichester, John Wiley.

Department of Health (2000). *Modernising NHS dentistry – implementing the NHS plan*. London, Department of Health.

Faculty of Dental Surgery (1991). *Clinical standards in general dental practice: self assessment manual and standards*. London, Faculty of Dental Surgery.

Locker, D. (1988). Measuring oral health: a conceptual framework. *Community Dental Health*, **5**, 3–18.

Sheiham, A. and Spencer, J. (1997). Health needs assessment. In *Community oral health* (ed. C. Pine), pp. 39–54. Oxford, Wright.

22 Health economics

CONTENTS

By the end of this chapter you should be able to:

- Understand the reasons why health economics are part of modern health services.
- Understand the main types of economic analyses.
- Have an overview of work done in dentistry.

This chapter links with:
- Introduction to the principles of public health (Chapter 1).
- Determinants of health (Chapter 2).
- Overview of epidemiology (Chapter 5).
- Evidence-based dentistry (Chapter 7).
- Planning dental services (Chapter 21).

INTRODUCTION

Health economics can be defined as:

The study of the application of economic theory to health and health care.

Why should economic theory have any relationship to health and health care? Clinicians will often state that they make their decisions based on their clinical judgement (what is best for the patient in front of them) and that they should not be influenced by concerns over money. Is this view entirely valid?

Despite the improvements in health seen in the majority of countries, costs of health care have continued to rise above the general rate of inflation (Schieber 1987). This is due to a number of factors, such as the price of materials, personnel wages, and the use of more advanced technology. However, there is little evidence that the increased spending has contributed to better health (Abel-Smith 1996). McKinlay and McKinlay 1977 demonstrated that there was little relationship between the increase in the expenditure in the United States and mortality when the effect of 11 infectious diseases had been removed (see fig. 22.1). Health will not be improved just by spending more money on health care.

However, increased spending may not necessarily be inappropriate. If better health resulted then society might well accept the rise in costs. Society does, though, seem to have problems with the growing expenditure on health care and governments have failed to increase health expenditure to meet changing needs or demands, both of which have increased, for many

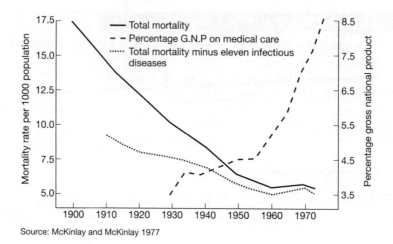

Source: McKinlay and McKinlay 1977

Fig. 22.1 Age- and sex-adjusted mortality rates for the United States (1900–73) (including and excluding eleven major infectious diseases) contrasted with the proportion of Gross National Product expended on medical care. (Reproduced from Locker 1989. See Permissions.)

reasons, over the years. For example, technological developments have led to the ability to provide more treatment that may be more expensive. The increase in the prevalence in chronic diseases means that more people may demand more treatment in order to alleviate their symptoms.

Health economics has been applied to answering questions about the justification for using resources. A key concept is the *opportunity cost of a programme*, which can be described as the value of the resource when it is put to its best alternative use (Cunningham 2000). Economic analysis compares the opportunity cost with the improvement in health produced by a particular programme. Essentially a comparison is made of the alternatives and the costs and consequences of the alternatives (Lewis and Morgan 1994).

Health economics is, therefore, about resource management – what is affordable and desirable and what is not. When resources are scarce, decisions need to be made as to how best to allocate them. If resources are scarce then it is usually not possible to provide all care that is desired and some form of rationing is introduced.

DISCUSSION POINTS

Why might rationing be controversial within the health system?

WHEN IS ECONOMIC EVALUATION APPROPRIATE?

Consider the question: 'What is the best way of preventing dental caries?' Is it through using self-applied fluoride toothpaste or professionally applied

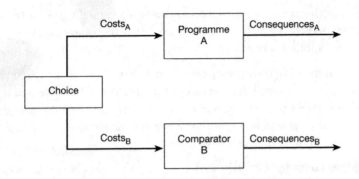

Fig. 22.2 Comparative analysis of alternative courses of action in economic evaluation. (Reproduced from Drummond *et al.* 1997. See Permissions.)

fluoride rinses? These are very wide questions and there are a variety of answers. Does the question mean: which produces the greatest reduction in dental caries, or which is more acceptable to the public, or which is cheaper? There are many factors involved in answering these questions and economic evaluation should be considered as only one. Drummond *et al.* (1997) stated that economic evaluation should come after three other questions are asked of any intervention. These questions are:

- Can the intervention work?
- Does it work in a real-life situation?
- Does it reach those whom it is meant to reach?

It can thus be seen that health economics should be closely related to evidenced-based dentistry. Once the effectiveness of an intervention has been determined, economics may help in deciding between two or more interventions.

In order to make comparisons a considerable amount of information is needed. Firstly, it is necessary to identify whether there are two alternatives that can be compared and is illustrated in Fig. 2.2. Only by having as complete information as possible can a full range of analysis be undertaken. Economic analyses are concerned with two major factors. Drummond stated that it deals with the inputs or costs, and the outputs or consequences of actions. The second factor that is involved is an element of choice. Which of the two interventions will give the best outcome?

INPUTS

To undertake an evaluation the inputs or costs need to be identified. These are the resources consumed and can be divided into three types. They are:

Direct costs Largely in the health sector, and include salaries and consumables. In a fluoride rinse programme the costs would be of the rinse used and the health care personnel involved. However, it might be that the rinse was supervised by teachers in schools and then the salary costs would be incurred by another sector.

Indirect costs Also known as production losses, these occur when someone cannot attend work while receiving therapy. Travelling time and loss of time from school are other examples. The indirect costs would be higher if someone had to attend a surgery for a fluoride application compared with applying the fluoride themselves at home.

Intangible costs Include pain and suffering, and are difficult to measure. Sociodental indicators have been developed as a way of trying to measure the impact and cost of dental diseases (Locker 1989). In oral diseases, where the majority of disease processes are chronic, these costs may be large.

OUTPUTS

The changes in health also need to be measured. The measures that are used depend upon the type of analysis that is being undertaken. Three types of unit are used and they are:
- *Natural units*; for example tooth surfaces saved are used in cost-effectiveness studies.
- *Utility measures*; for example, quality-adjusted life years are used in cost-utility studies. These are calculated by using life-years gained by an intervention weighted by the values that people place on different states of health.
- *Monetary units* are used in cost-benefit analyses.

TYPES OF ECONOMIC ANALYSIS

The types of analysis are summarized in Fig. 22.3 by Drummond *et al.*, 1997.

Cost effectiveness

Cost effectiveness analysis can be used to compare any intervention with any other intervention, provided the same outcome measure is used. In dentistry it would be a very appropriate methodology to use when comparing different types of preventive treatments. The unit of measurement would be tooth surfaces saved per year. Thus it is possible to compare different types of intervention, for example fissure sealants with fluoridated toothpaste, where the outcome (here number of tooth surfaces) can be measured in the same unit. The level of effectiveness is different as are the costs, but a cost per unit saved can be calculated and comparison can therefore be made. In this case an attempt is made to express all the outcomes in a monetary unit.

Type of Study	Measurement/ valuation of costs in both alternatives	Identification of consequences	Measurement/ valuation of consequences
Cost-minimization analysis	Dollars	Identical in all relevant respects	None
Cost-effectiveness analysis	Dollars	Single effect of interest, common to both alternatives, but achieved to different degrees	Natural units (e.g. life-years gained, disability-days saved, points of blood pressure reduction, etc.)
Cost-utility analysis	Dollars	Single or multiple effects, not necessarily common to both alternatives	Healthy years or (more often) quality-adjusted life-years
Cost-benefit analysis	Dollars	Single or multiple effects, not necessarily common to both alternatives	Dollars

Fig. 22.3 Measurement of costs and consequences in economic evaluation. (Reproduced from Drummond *et al.* 1997. See Permissions.)

However, it can be difficult to express, for example, the number of days lost from work as a financial amount. Sometimes it is appropriate to do this, and it can then lead to a ratio of costs to benefits, and thus disparate results or multiple outcome measures can be combined. This type of analysis means that all types of benefit are expressed in monetary units. The question needs to be posed, however, as to whether or not it is reasonable to express some benefits, for example reduction in pain, as a monetary value. This has led to the development of cost utility analysis.

Cost utility

To overcome the concerns of expressing all benefits in terms of money an alternative measure is used and that is the concept of utility. Utility means the preferences people or society have for a set of health outcomes. Different people value different health states in different ways. Imagine the situation where two people suffer from lingual anaesthesia following the removal of a lower third molar. One person is a tea taster while the other is a nurse. The impact upon the life of the tea taster is going to be significant in terms of her ability to function at work. She is therefore going to rate the effect of the treatment markedly worse on a scale of 0 (dead) to 1 (perfect health) than the nurse as it will interfere with her work far more. Utility analysis allows for a quality of life measure to be incorporated as well as the costs and outcomes in different programmes. The usual outcome measure in which all of these values are expressed is quality-adjusted life years. Some work has also been done using the measure quality-adjusted tooth years. The outcomes of this type of analysis are usually expressed as cost per life year gained.

Cost benefit

Sometimes it is desirable to compare interventions with more than one outcome, or where it is not possible to express the outcome in the same unit. For example, it may be considered desirable to compare the cost per surface saved *and* the reduction in the amount of toothache for both interventions. There are now four measures which need to be looked at. If one intervention is not clearly in the lead then it is difficult to compare the two interventions and it may be desirable to combine the measures into one overall benefit.

Cost minimization

In health economics the term cost minimization has a specific meaning, but it also has another meaning in everyday use. It is important to understand which meaning is implied. Economic cost-minimization analyses are a specific type of cost-effectiveness study. The outcomes of the programmes being compared are tested through controlled clinical trials, ideally running concurrently. If the clinical outcomes of the interventions are the same then only the costs need to be compared. The intervention with the lowest costs would be selected, but these analyses are rare as the outcomes between programmes are rarely identical.

The common use of the term refers to reductions in expenditure. For example, a hospital that needs to balance its budget may refer to the closure of a ward or the alteration of services as 'cost minimization'. This is not an economic analysis.

HOW HEALTH ECONOMICS DIFFERS FROM OTHER ECONOMIC EVALUATIONS OF GOODS AND SERVICES

In economic theory the consumer has a central position in the evaluation of goods and services. It is not possible to *trade* health but it is possible to buy and sell health services (McGuire *et al.* 1988). Economic evaluation of health care differs from other economic evaluations of goods and services in four key aspects (Cunningham 2000; McGuire *et al.* 1988; Mooney 1992):

1. There is an assumption that a consumer makes a choice after receiving information. However, consumers are not always able to collect or process information in relation to health care.
2. The person providing the information is usually the supplier of the health care. This does not happen in other fields.

3. There is an assumption that once health care is consumed benefits in terms of improvements in health status will occur.
4. It is assumed that health is the only outcome of value for consumers. Consumers do not voluntarily engage in consuming health care. However, it has been argued that this may not be the case for dentistry (Cunningham 2000).

HEALTH ECONOMICS IN DENTISTRY

One of the major problems in dentistry is taking the results of a clinical trial and trying to turn that into a lifetime benefit from an intervention. For example, if it is known that using fluoridated toothpaste will reduce carious surfaces by of 0.8 surfaces per year in children aged 12 to 15, what will be the benefits over the next 15 years compared with restoring these surfaces?

DISCUSSION POINTS

Discuss the example in the previous paragraph. Start by making a list of inputs and outputs as described above, and then try to make a list of the factors which would be included.

Some of the problems with extending this example beyond the 3 years would include taking account of factors such as the changes in caries incidence over this time, the failure rate of restorations, and the value people place on restored surfaces compared with sound surfaces. Many of these factors are just not known. There is evidence both on how long restorations last in clinical trials and how frequently they are replaced in real-life situations (Chadwick *et al.* 1999), but these two figures are very different. When this happens it is sensible to repeat the analyses using different estimates of inputs; this is known as undertaking sensitivity analyses. The likelihood of the accuracy of these estimates depends upon the validity of the data, which in some cases may be as little as an educated guess! These factors need to be acknowledged in the reporting of the results. Particularly in an example where you are trying to predict the life-long benefit of a preventive example, the results will become more speculative the further from the clinical trial results you move.

CONCLUSION

Health economics can be a useful tool to help assess the value of different interventions. In dentistry the number of robust studies using these techniques is relatively small and generally limited to preventive techniques. As with many tools, health economics is limited by the quality of the data available to put into the analyses. Health economics cannot provide a complete answer as to which intervention to use but can provide very useful data which will inform a decision.

REFERENCES

Abel-Smith, B. (1996). *The escalation of health care costs: how did we get there? Health Care Reform. The will to change.* Paris, OECD, 17–30.

Chadwick, B., Dummer, P. Dunstan, F., *et al.* (1999). *A systematic review of the longevity of dental restorations.* York, NHS Centre for Reviews and Dissemination, University of York.

Cunningham, S. J. (2000). Economic Evaluation of health care-is it important to us? *British Dental Journal,* **188**, 250–6.

Drummond, M., Stoddart, G. O'Brien, B. J., *et al.* (1997). *Methods for the economic evaluation of health care programmes.* Oxford, Oxford University Press.

Lewis, J. M. and Morgan, M. V. (1994) A critical review of methods for the economic evaluation of fissure sealants. *Community Dental Health,* **11**, 79–82.

Locker, D. (1989). *An introduction to behavioural science and dentistry.* London, Routledge.

McGuire, A., Henderson, J., and Mooney, G. (1988) *The economics of healthcare-an introduction text,* London, Routledge and Kegan Paul.

McKinlay, J. and McKinlay, S. (1977). The questionable contribution of medical measures to the decline in mortality in the United States in the twentieth century. *Millbank Memorial Fund Quarterly,* **55**, 405–28.

Schieber, G. J. (1987). *Financing and delivering health care: a comparative analysis of OECD countries.* Paris, OECD, 54–9.

FURTHER READING

Drummond, M., Stoddart, G. O'Brien, B. J., *et al.* (1997). *Methods for the economic evaluation of health care programmes.* Oxford, Oxford University Press.

Mooney, G. (1992). *Economics, medicine and health care.* London, Harvester Wheatsheaf.

23 Problems with health services

CONTENTS

By the end of this chapter you should be able to:

- Describe the common problems with health care delivery.
- Define the term 'access to care' / 'barriers to care'.
- Briefly outline how the barriers to care might be overcome for disadvantaged groups.
- Define the term inequality and its relationship to the receipt of care and experience of poor health.

This chapter links with:
- Introduction to the principles of public health (Chapter 1).
- Evidence-based dentistry (Chapter 7).
- The structure of the NHS in the UK (Chapter 18).
- The structure of dental services in the UK (Chapter 19).
- Planning health services (Chapter 21).

INTRODUCTION

Earlier chapters have highlighted the influence the medical model of health has had on both the philosophy of health care and the structures devised to deliver health care. The overriding influences of the medical model are the downstream focus on treatment of disease and the communication gap caused by differing concepts of health held by lay people and health professionals. Plamping (1988) has summarized the problems of health care delivery (Box 23.1) at the macro level, that is, at the level of structures and policy. Chapter 18 has described some of the specific problems with healthcare in the UK. In this chapter we shall also look at some of the problems with health services at the level of the user and the provider of health care.

COMMON PROBLEMS WITH HEALTH CARE DELIVERY

Chapter 1 discussed the limitations of the medical model of health. The legacy has been treatment-focused services dominated by health professionals. Resources are spent on high technology medicine and hospitals, while programmes to prevent disease are poorly supported and resourced. There is an expectation of a magic bullet for every health problem, yet most chronic diseases have no cure. People learn to adapt and cope with their illness. While treatment of disease is an important part of health care, it should be

Box 23.1 Common problems with health care delivery

- Insufficient resources.
- Insufficient emphasis on prevention and public health.
- Unclear goals.
- Inadequate organization and management.
  Poor planning.
  Administration not unified.
  Little emphasis on evaluation.
- Inequality of distribution of services regionally.
- Failure in manpower planning and use of ancillary workers.
- Inequitable access for people in certain localities and those with disabilities, and for older and socially disadvantaged people.
- Method of payment of dentists does not promote high professional standards.
- Lack of public accountability and public involvement.
- Dental training is not oriented to health service goals (attachment to a medical rather than a social model of health.
- Dental research is not sufficiently oriented to health care needs and prevention.
- Unclear strategies for implementing policies.
- Access problems.

(Plamping 1988)

DISCUSSION POINTS

Look at the problems identified in Box 23.1. Think of examples of each 'problem' you have heard about or experienced personally.

linked to an appropriate mix of care (teaching and supporting people to cope with chronic illness and disability), cure, and prevention.

Health care consumes huge amounts of resources. The dominance of the medical model and the race to build large hospitals and find ever better medicines and better technology blinded people to the important question 'Are people healthier as a result of this spending on health care?' It would appear not to be the case. Consider the work of McKeown and Cochrane, and the findings of the Black report, discussed in Chapter 1. Deciding whether health has improved is complex. First, health has to be defined; secondly, there is a need to choose an indicator of health status which will allow the measurement of change; and thirdly, any change in health status needs to be linked to an antecedent health care intervention within very strict limiting criteria. The evidence from the Black report and the more recent Acheson Report (1998) suggests that despite all the money spelt on health care in the UK huge health inequality still exists.

A big problem with much health care delivery is that programmes do not define the health goals that need to be achieved by the programme. Put simply, *If we don't know where we want to be, how do we know when we get there?* The health goals for a programme should be specific, measurable, appropriate, realistic, time-related, and important (SMARTI). They should also be challenging so there is an incentive for health care providers and users to change.

Despite ever-increasing spending on health care, it will never be possible to satisfy every health care need and want. For example, it is recognized that urban areas are often better provided for than rural areas, hospital-based health care consumes more resources than community-based services, and people living in deprived communities with greater health need have less doctors and dentists than richer areas with less health care need (Tudor Hart 1971). Uncomfortable choices and rationing has to take place in allocating health care resources, and ideally should be based on the greatest health need rather than who have the loudest voices.

The dominance of the medical model has meant that the users of health care (the patients) are often seen by professionals as passive recipients. Yet the consumers pay for every part of the health service, including the training of health professionals. Lack of accountability and poor communication between provider and consumer of health care is one of the biggest issues in health care delivery. People frequently complain that they feel rushed in the surgery, their treatment is poorly explained, and their concerns are not adequately dealt with.

ACCESS PROBLEMS

Access to health care is a complex issue, which can have two aspects. The first aspect relates to the factors which influence whether a person will make contact with health services. These are factors which have sociological and psychological explanations, and examples include how culture can affect a person's response to symptoms and use of services and also how people's beliefs, attitudes, expectations, and definitions of sickness can affect service use. The second aspect of access relates to the fit between the health care service and the clients, assuming the latter have overcome cultural and psychological issues and have decided to use health care. Penchansky and Thomas (1981) considered the problems of health service use under five headings (see Box 23.2). They use the term 'access' problems to describe the difficulties experienced with service use.

Availability of services

This refers to how well distributed health services are; for example, the ratio of dentists to the population in a locality. It has been well described that

---

Box 23.2 Access problems

- Availability of services.
- Accessibility of services.
- Affordability of services.
- Acceptability of services.
- Accommodation of services.

(Penchansky and Thomas 1981)

---

doctors like to set up practices in middle class areas where need for such services is small. Thus we have an abundance of practices in middle class areas and a small number in more deprived areas where needs are greater. This paradox was described by Tudor-Hart as the *inverse care law*. Another consequence of the perception of the availability of services is the impact on the uptake of care. If it is perceived that services are limited then demand for care becomes suppressed.

DISCUSSION POINTS

What things are worth paying for?

What services are of value to you, and how do you make that judgement?

Accessibility of services

The accessibility of services has two dimensions. The first is about location: how far you have to travel to the nearest dental practice. For example, what is local transport like if you are not a car owner? The second aspect is a spatial dimension: whether a person can physically access the premises. For example, an older person with arthritis would find climbing stairs to reach a dental surgery a significant barrier to visiting that practice.

Affordability of services

It is well known that having to pay for dental treatment can act as a barrier to people using dental services. This is true in the UK even in groups where dental treatment is subsidized by the state. Of course, in addition to the direct costs of dental treatment there are some indirect costs that people include in the equation about whether 'it is worth' having dental treatment. Examples of such indirect costs are: having to take time off work, having to pay travel costs, and having to pay for child-care while at the dentist. Some groups will suffer greater disadvantage depending on how they are paid. Low income workers are usually paid by the hour, and the cost to them of taking time off work is greater than to someone on a salary.

Acceptability of services

Users and providers of health services have expectations about how services should look and be. These expectations are not always shared. Providers want to attract to their practice 'patients' who speak the language, pay on time, behave well in the waiting room, and enhance the image of the practice. Users would like to be made to feel welcome in the practice and to feel information was easy to find, and they would like to be dealt with professionally but treated as an individual. The acceptability of patients to a practice is an important issue: a dental study of homeless people in London found that they would rather use an older shabbier dental hospital than the newly built more local dental hospital, because they perceived that older hospital was more accepting of their appearance and circumstances.

Accommodation

This refers to the way in which care is provided in terms of opening hours, emergency visits, late night clinics, waiting times, and ease of getting an appointment. Many people feel that a drop-in dental service would be ideal. Such services are being piloted in the general medical and dental services.

The Penchansky and Thomas framework is very useful for identifying the structural problems in the organization of health care, but it ignores the behavioural science explanation of access.

TOWARDS A NEW CONCEPTUALIZATION OF ACCESS

A recent review by the Department of Dental Public Health (2001) at Guys and Kings Trust, King's College London, has highlighted the limitations of existing definitions and models of access. Limitations were identified as:

- Lack of clarity.
- The roles of factors that operate at several stages in the process of access are considered as separate events. These events are then measured in isolation and their interlinkage and interdependence is ignored.
- There is an artificial split between gaining entry and using a service, so that 'gaining entry as defined by a registration rate' is given equal importance to actually using a service and using it appropriately.

A new approach to access has been advocated that defines access as part of a general theoretical framework. Access is related to health rather than service use. Access is defined as 'the experience and command of socially produced resources for health, where command is the expression of a person's experience' (Department of Dental Public Health 2001). Command denotes the person's capacity to command resources by demanding and using planning services, and participating in health promotion (Department of Dental Public Health 2001). Figure 23.1 provides a preliminary model of

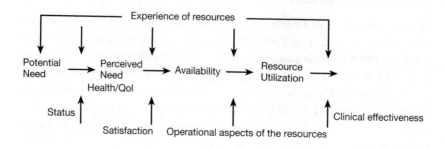

Fig. 23.1 Model of access. (Reproduced from Department of Dental Public Health 2001 with permission. See Permissions.)

this definition. Access is the interaction of three broad groups of determinants:

- the individual and group experience of resources;
- the operational aspects of the resources;
- the effectiveness of the particular way in which they are used.

The interactions may occur at one or more stages in the access to the resources. They create health needs and influence the perception of need, the availability and utilization of resources, and the outcomes of that utilization.

ACCESS PROBLEMS AND DENTAL CARE

In 1985 Finch examined the reasons why people did not use dental services regularly, and she used the term 'barriers to the receipt of dental care'. Her findings are reproduced in Box 23.3. The terms 'access to care' and 'barriers to care' are both used in the literature but essentially mean the same thing.

Patient expectations in developed countries have changed in the last 50 years. In the UK in the 1940s replacement of the natural dentition with dentures was a normal occurrence for people in their forties. Now people expect to keep their natural dentition for life. Despite a heavily subsidized dental service in the UK, people still cite fear and cost as the two most important barriers to seeking care (Finch *et al.* 1988). In 1998 lack of information and openness continued to be a common complaint about dental care in the UK, and there appeared to be a diminution of trust between dentists and patients (Centre for Dental Service Studies 1998).

APPROPRIATE SERVICE USE

The appropriate use of health services is a complex issue. People may have very valid reasons for using services in a way that health professionals may

---

Box 23.3 Barriers to the receipt of dental care

Two main barriers

- Fear and cost of dental treatment.

Other barriers

- Reception and waiting room procedures.
- Loss of control.
- Personality of the dentist
- Clinical smell.
- Hearing the sounds of dental treatment.
- White coats and bright lights.
- Feeling vulnerable in dental chair.
- Getting treated like you are a mouth.
- Travel time, time off work.

(Finch et al. *1988)*

DISCUSSION POINTS

Imagine you are on holiday alone, backpacking. You visit a country whose language you do not speak. You fall ill with a tummy bug. You need to see a doctor urgently.

What are your concerns about this?
What information will you need?
How and where will you get it?
How does all this make you feel?

Now return to your answers and apply the Penchansky and Thomas framework to explore the barriers you might face in this situation.

---

not advise. The conflict over what is considered to be appropriate use of dental services draws us back to lay and health professional communication problems. Because lay people have different expectations and different concepts of health, their use of health services will reflect these differences. Consider the issue of regular attendance at the dentist. In the UK the accepted advice over the years has been regular attendance every 6 months. But given the decline in decay rates amongst young people, this is no longer and appropriate recommendation. As people become more aware of oral health issues many are choosing not to attend regularly (that is at 6-monthly intervals), because they know from past experience they need very little oral health care. Guidance on what is regular attendance must depend on the individual, their oral health problems (if any), and their life circumstances.

DISCUSSION POINTS

What advice about regular attendance would you give to a healthy 23-year-old with a DMFT of 2 and good oral hygiene?

What advice about regular attendance would you give to a mother with two children under five, both of whom have decayed teeth?

What advice about regular attendance would you give to a 60-year-old man with a heavily restored dentition and evidence of attachment loss?

What were the reasons for your recommendations?

DISADVANTAGED GROUPS

Many different groups in societies have difficulties in accessing dental services. Most of these groups have diverse problems which bring about disadvantage, but what they do share is a common experience of access problems. Some disadvantaged groups are now well recognized and efforts have been made to make services more flexible to their particular needs. Examples include people with learning difficulties, people with physical handicap, elderly people who are housebound, people living with HIV and AIDS, and people such as lone parents living in poverty.

The small grid in Table 23.1 examines some of the structural barriers (Penchansky and Thomas 1981) certain disadvantaged groups face in accessing dental care. These are just some short examples. As an exercise, draw up a list of disadvantaged groups and try to describe an access problem or problems for each group. Then attempt to think of ways in which the problems might be overcome.

INEQUALITY

Inequality has been described as health differences which are avoidable, unnecessary, unjust, and unfair (Whitehead 1991). Inequalities have been observed between groups in a region and between different geographic regions in the same country. Inequality has been described in every type of political and social system worldwide. In order to assess an inequality we must first judge the situation against the background or context of what is happening in society generally. For example, while dental decay declined in the UK in all social classes between 1983 and 1993, the gap in experience of dental decay has widened between 12–15-year-olds from skilled households (who had improved most) and children from semi-skilled and unskilled households (who had improved least). See Chapter 6 for a more detailed summary of oral health in the UK and oral health inequality.

Table 23.1 Structural barriers to receiving dental care

Disadvantage	Main problem in using a health service	Additional problems in using a health service	Solution to problem
People with learning difficulties	Communication problems	Surgery may deter clients because other patients in waiting room are fearful of them	Education of dental reception staff Development of appropriate advocacy skills in carers of and with people with learning difficulties
People with physical handicap	Cannot access health service because of stairs	May need specialized transport to get to dental surgery	Identify list of local practices that have ground-floor access; arrange for appropriate transport Provide a domiciliary service
Elderly people who are housebound	Cannot leave the house		
Lone parents on low income	Cannot afford childcare	Subsidized dental care may not be well advertised	Identify local list of dentists who welcome children in waiting room and provide subsidized dental care

Box 23.4 The determinants of health inequality

1. Natural, genetic. or biological variation.
2. Health-damaging behaviour if freely chosen; for example participation in certain sports.
3. The transient health advantage when one group is the first to adopt a health-promoting behaviour which then becomes widespread; for example, placing babies on their backs to sleep to reduce risk of cot death.
4. Health-damaging behaviour, where the choice of lifestyle is severely restricted; for example, living in damp housing.
5. Exposure to unhealthy, stressful, living and working conditions; for example, miners and chronic lung disease.
6. Inadequate access to essential health and other public services; for example, homeless people.
7. Natural selection or health-related social mobility where there is a tendency for sick people to move down the social scale.

(Reproduced with permission from Whitehead 1991. See Permissions.)

Evidence suggests that disadvantaged groups have poorer survival chances and a greater experience of illness during their lifetime compared to more favoured groups.

So, what is the basis of the inequality and how may it be addressed? Whitehead (1991) has summarized the determinants of health inequality which are reproduced in Box 23.4.

When we analyse the first three determinants it is obvious that these inequalities are neither unnecessary, unjust, or unfair. But the latter four clearly are and need to be addressed. It is not feasible to devise strategies (which would include health promotion and the provision of health care services) to ensure everyone has the same standard of health and access to health care. Whitehead suggests we should be looking to achieve 'a fair distribution throughout the country based on health care needs and ease of access in each geographical area and the removal of barriers to access.'

In order to reduce health differentials, we must return to the principles of health promotion. By improving living conditions, providing supportive environments, and cultivating greater participation of lay people in decision-making, it is possible to considerably reduce the determinants of poor health.

At the micro-level, inequality exists in terms of the outcomes of health care and the quality of care received. Middle class people usually get more consultation time with their doctor and are more likely to get referred for secondary care. They are also more likely to avail themselves of preventive services.

QUALITY OF CARE AND EVIDENCE-BASED DENTISTRY

Previous chapters have highlighted the new emphasis on clinical governance and evidence-based dental care. In the UK, since the inception of the NHS in 1948 the method of remuneration has remained virtually unchanged. This is despite new developments in materials and preventive care. Various dental reports during the 1960s and 1970s expressed concerns about the treatment-only emphasis of NHS dental services. The fee-per-item method of remuneration was identified as a problem because it favoured active treatment and dentists were not paid for time they spent on prevention. A report in Scotland noted that, despite patients being regular attenders, they were still receiving large amounts of treatment and such treatment was being provided a relatively short time after a previous course of treatment. What was going wrong?

Elderton co-ordinated a large study in Scotland that essentially studied the impact the dental service had on people's oral health over a 5-year period. He found that the more often a patient changed dentist the more treatment was received, compared to patients who did not change their dentist (Elderton and Davies 1984). Over half of all amalgam restorations had failed two and a half years after placement, and 25% of treatment provided was for maintenance of existing restorative work (Elderton and Davies 1984). Dentists were only paid per item of treatment and thus the incentive was to undertake active treatment.

Elderton (1986, 1997) linked these findings to previous work he had undertaken on cavity preparation and new work which had shown that the caries process can be halted. He concluded that dentists were using an outdated diagnosis and treatment philosophy. Rather than the 'if in doubt fill' philosophy in vogue at the time, he advocated the 'watch and wait' approach. He argued that an early carious lesion could arrest if the diet was changed and fluorides were applied. Thus the tooth's entrance into the 'restorative cycle' would be delayed. The restorative cycle was a term he used to describe how, once a tooth was filled, it was condemned to replacement and an ever-increasing filling size, until it eventually required extraction.

This was probably one of the first examples of introducing an evidence base to dentistry, though it was not called that at the time. It is an example of how important it is to constantly update and appraise clinical interventions and treatments. The compulsory introduction of peer review and continuing professional education schemes in 2000 has made the improving and maintaining of quality standards part of a dentist's requirements for registration. Clinical governance is being integrated into the structure of public funded health care systems in the UK. It is anticipated that all these measures will improve the quality and evidence base of health care for patients.

> **Box 23.5** Ethical nature of the client-provider encounter
>
> • Confidentiality.
> • Placing best interest of patients first.
> • Ensuring skill and competence.
> • Ensuring communication and trust.

ETHICS

A detailed discussion of this topic is beyond the scope of this text but a few aspects will be described insofar as they relate to the micro-aspects of the problems of health care delivery.

A dentist is obliged to maintain high standards of competency and experience, as has been discussed briefly above and on p. 260.

An important ethical consideration is ensuring confidentiality and trust. We noted at the beginning of the chapter that the influence of the medical model has led to differing concepts of health, expectations of health, and use of health services amongst dentists and lay people. A considerable amount of work needs to be done to close this communication gap. As holders of the body of knowledge dentists have a duty to explain options and costs of treatment, listen to patients' concerns, and ensure informed consent before they undertake dental treatment.

At the micro-level of the patient and the provider, a dentist has responsibility to ensure the ethical nature of the client–provider encounter (see Box 23.5). As an exercise, take each responsibility and consider how you ensure they are implemented in your own working situation.

CONCLUSIONS

The primary purpose of health care is to relieve pain and suffering, restore and maintain physical, psychological, and social functioning, and improve the quality of life. Within the UK, greater accountability is now required from commissioners and providers of health care to achieve these aims. The problems with health care delivery can occur at both a micro- and a macro-level of operation and require a whole-system approach to their solution. One such whole-system approach is the Alma-Ata Declaration as outlined in Chapter 1. The key features of this approach are worth stating again: equitable distribution; focus on prevention; appropriate technology; multisectoral approach; community participation.

REFERENCES

Acheson, D. (1998). *Independent inquiry into inequalities in health report*. London, The Stationery Office.

Centre for Dental Services Studies (1998). *Consumers views of dental care*. York University.

Department of Dental Public Health (2001). *A new conceptualisation of access*. Guys and Kings Trust, King's College London.

Elderton, R. J. (1987). Preventively orientated restorations and restorative procedures. In *Positive dental prevention* (ed. R. J. Elderton), pp. 256–72. Heinemann, London.

Elderton, R. (1996). The future of dentistry: treating restorative dentistry to health. *British Dental Journal*, **181**, 220–5.

Elderton, R. J. and Davies, J. A. (1984). Restorative dental treatment in the General Dental Service in Scotland. *British Dental Journal*, **157**, 196–200.

Finch, H., Keegar, J., Ward, K., and Sanyal Sen, B. (1988). *Barriers to the receipt of dental care*. British Dental Association, London.

Murray, C. J. L., Kawabata, K., and Valentine, N. (2001). People's experience versus people's expectations. *Health Affairs*, **20**, 21–4.

Penchansky, R. and Thomas, J. W. (1981). The concept of access: definition and relationship to consumer satisfaction. *Medical Care*, **1**, 127–40.

Plamping, D. (1988). The primary health care approach. Lecture notes, MSc in Dental Public Health. University College London.

Plamping, D. and Jacob-Casey, M. (1989). *The practice of primary dental care*. Wright, London.

Tudor Hart, J. (1971). The inverse care law. *Lancet*, **i**, 405–12.

Whitehead, M. (1991). The concepts and principles of equity and health. *Health Promotion International*, **6**, 217–26.

24 Dental organizations

CONTENTS

By the end of this chapter you should be able to:
- Outline the main dental organizations within the UK.
- Describe their functions.

This chapter links with:
The structure of dental services in the UK (Chapter 19)

INTRODUCTION

This chapter looks at the roles and functions of the main dental organizations, which all have up-to-date and well-maintained websites that include lists of current publications, policies, and news items. These are important sites and should be consulted to find any changes.

GENERAL DENTAL COUNCIL

http://www.gdc-uk.org
The dental profession in the UK is self-regulating, which means that it develops and implements its own policies and enforces its own standards. In order to practice dentistry it is necessary to register with the General Dental Council (GDC) and to pay an annual retention fee. The GDC is the statutory body (i.e. its responsibilities are laid down in law) charged with protecting the public by ensuring adherence to the Dentists Act. It is also responsible for dental education, the registration of dentists, auxiliaries, and specialist practitioners, professional conduct, and the health of dentists and dental auxiliaries.

The GDC's functions include the maintenance of the UK Dentists Register and the Rolls of Dental Auxiliaries, the promotion of the high standards of dental education at all stages, and high standards of professional conduct among dentists. A register is published annually, listing the dental care worker's initial qualification date, along with their subsequent qualifications.

The present GDC was constituted by the 1984 Dentists Act, although it was created in 1956. Prior to this, the GDC's functions were administered by the Dental Board of the UK, which was constituted by the Dentists Act of 1921. Until the changes in 1984, the Board and the dental profession remained subject to the overriding control of the General Medical Council.

The GDC is made up of 50 members; 18 are elected by the profession, 17 are nominated by dental schools or the Royal Colleges, and 6 are lay members. Other representatives include the Chief Dental Officers of each of the four countries of the UK, three members of the General Medical Council, and a dental auxiliary.

The GDC's educational functions relate to the inspection and approval of courses for training dentists and other dental staff. Dental schools are visited to ensure that adequate standards are met and that the degree awarded is suitable as a qualification for registration as a dentist. It has the power to declare that a qualification is unsuitable, but this is not done without warning. The GDC also determines the basic curriculum and this is published (General Dental Council 1997a). It makes similar prescriptions for the training of hygienists and therapists.

A major function of the GDC is to, where necessary, discipline dentists. There are three stages to the consideration of complaints and convictions. The evidence is considered first by the president, then the Preliminary Proceedings Committee, and finally the Professional Conduct Committee. If the president considers that there is evidence of serious professional misconduct the case is passed to the Preliminary Proceedings Committee. This committee asks all parties to submit written evidence and then decides whether there is a case to answer. If there is, then the case moves to the Professional Conduct Committee, which usually meets twice a year.

The Professional Conduct Committee meets in public and follows the same procedures as any British court. A legal assessor is present and advises on points of law. The GDC's case is presented by a barrister and the dentist is usually similarly represented. The standard of proof is the same as that in a criminal court. If a dentist is found guilty, a variety of conclusions may be reached. A decision may be delayed for one year while reports on the dentist's progress are received, a warning may be given, or the dentist's registration may be suspended or erased. A dentist has the right of appeal to the Judicial Committee of the Privy Council. The decision of the Professional Conduct Committee does not take effect for 28 days, unless the committee feels there is a need to protect the public (General Dental Council 1997b).

As a separate process to disciplinary procedures, the GDC may take action if it suspects a dentist has impaired ability to practice dentistry due to a health problem. The dentist may be asked to have a medical examination and recommendations may be made.

DISCUSSION POINT

What are the advantages and disadvantages of a profession being self-regulating? Start by thinking of the conflicts of interest that might arise and the specialist knowledge available.

The future

The GDC has proposed major reforms to its constitution in response to the need to increase lay representation. The structure of the Council will change, as will the disciplinary procedures. Readers should consult the GDC website and the website of this book.

LOCAL DENTAL COMMITTEES

Local Dental Committees (or LDCs) are statutory bodies established in 1948. Under NHS legislation health authorities are required to consult with LDCs on matters of local dental interest. Membership of the LDC is by election. LDCs will also make nominations to, or be consulted about membership of certain committees and offer advice in four broad areas of dental activity: provision of dental services, complaints, advice on regulatory matters, and education.

The LDC has an input into provision of dental services at a local level by advising the health authority on the needs for services; for example, specialist services or perhaps establishing a service to provide out of hours cover for registered patients. The LDC helps the health authority deal with complaints and dentists implement guidance on health and safety legislation. The committee would also advises on educational issues such as the appointment of vocational trainers and clinical audit and peer review activity.

THE DENTAL PROTECTION SOCIETIES

http://www.the-mdu.com/ and http://www.mps.org.uk

The Medical Protection Society and the Dental Defence Union are international associations run for doctors and dentists to provide medico-legal services. It is important to note that there are also insurance companies that offer similar services. The defence organizations offer ethical and legal advice on a large range of topics, not only with regard to complaints. They offer professional indemnity for the award of costs and damages for medical negligence. Health authorities and employing trusts carry insurance for medical negligence but this does not cover all risks for the individual practitioner, and does not cover general practice. The Medical Protection Society lists the following functions on its web site:
- Negligence claims, including indemnity for damages and costs.
- Medical (Dental) Council proceedings.
- Health authority/board and hospital inquiries.
- Disciplinary proceedings for alleged professional misconduct or incompetence.
- Inquests.
- Complaints.
- Criminal matters arising from professional practice.

BRITISH DENTAL ASSOCIATION

http://www.bda-dentistry.org.uk

The professional association for dentists is the British Dental Association (BDA), which states that it aims to promote the interests of members, advance the science, arts, and ethics of dentistry, and to improve the nation's oral health.

The BDA acts as a professional organization to its members and to the public. This means that it has a variety of functions:

- It negotiates pay and conditions of service with the appropriate pay bodies.
- It provides an information service for its members.
- It acts as a lobby group.
- It promotes the profession to the public.
- It supports research aimed to improve oral health.
- It provides educational courses to maintain the standards of its members.

It is responsible for representing the views of members both to government and the public, but it also acts as an advocate for promoting policies that will improve the oral health of the nation. For example, it has accredited some products that are known to be effective at reducing dental caries.

The committee organization of the BDA is based both on a local structure, where all sections of the profession meet together, and a professional structure based on the different types of practising dentists. There are groups for hospital dentists, for general practitioners, for community dentists, and for university teachers and research workers.

REFERENCES

General Dental Council (1997a). *The first five years*. London, General Dental Council.
General Dental Council (1997b). *Maintaining standards: guidance to dentists on professional and personal conduct. London*. General Dental Council.

Index

training of dentists 273–4, 280, 281, 283, 295, 296, 344
traumatic dental injuries
aetiology 237
epidemiology 100, 102, 236
impact 236–7
limitations of treatment 238
preventive options 238
public health approaches to prevention 233–9
treatment index 82
trends in oral health 89–106
true negatives 56
true positives 56

unmet need 39

validity 71
victim blaming approach 27, 138

whole-population approach to prevention 50–2, 141, 213